DICTIONARY OF FRENCH MEDICAL TERMS

With an introduction to the French medical system

FRENCH–ENGLISH
ENGLISH–FRENCH

Edited by Richard Whiting

summersdale

DICTIONARY OF FRENCH MEDICAL TERMS

Text by Richard Whiting

Summersdale Publishers Ltd
46 West Street
Chichester
West Sussex
PO19 1RP
UK

www.summersdale.com

Printed and bound in Great Britain

ISBN: 1-84024-575-1
ISBN 13: 978-1-84024-575-2

CONTENTS

PREFACE

France is generally recognised as the best medical service provider in the world and has almost twice as many doctors per person as in the UK. It is a big country and while you may find a doctor or pharmacist with whom you can communicate with in English, by consulting the Internet or obtaining a list from American and British consulates, they will not necessarily be near where you are holidaying or regularly visit or where you've decided to settle. Truly bi-lingual doctors are extremely rare and there are just approximately 100 British nationals who practise in France.

The scope of health care and entitlements is wide and somewhat sophisticated in its complexity and the considerable advances in medicine in recent years mean that medical vocabulary increases all the time. (Radiology, to take a simple example, is no longer confined to the examination and interpretation of X-ray plates).While French *spécialistes* can no doubt make themselves understood talking shop with their British counterparts at international conferences, the French layman, and his British equivalent when in France, are increasingly at a disadvantage.

This book explains, therefore, for visitors and new residents to France how the medical system works, before going on to the main dictionary which is in two sections. Firstly, health service and administrative terms, and then terms and descriptions useful for seeing GPs, dentists, oculists, opticians, physiotherapists, chiropodists and other specialists as well as pharmacists and blood test laboratorists. It will also be beneficial for reading and understanding medical correspondance and check-up results. (Since 2002 everyone in France is legally entitled to access all information held by doctors and hospitals concerning their health.) Throughout the two dictionary sections, where the translation into English is considered too technical, or if the original medical word in English is considered too technical, a simple explanation follows so that recourse to another reference book should not be necessary. Abbreviations that the reader may encounter and what they stand for in French are indicated, and translated. Vaccinations, medicines, diet, hygiene, health care, medical comfort and orthopaedic products are also included. The dictionary is followed by a phrase-book and useful questions for situations most likely to be encountered in emergencies, hospitals and pharmacies, at the doctor and the dentist.

My thanks go to Dr Pierre Agin, consultant and head of the medical imaging department at Hôpital Font-Pré, Toulon, who ensured that no appropriate area of medical information was omitted and to my wife Nicole who checked the French genders, translations and spellings. Monsieur M. Brunet, pharmacist at the Pharmacie de Bucarin, Six-Fours, was also most helpful in providing information on certain drugs and medicines.

Keep *A Dictionary of French Medical Terms* handy. It will help you get the best out of the first-class service and care available and avoid any misunderstandings.

Richard Whiting

Disclaimer

Every effort has been made to ensure that the information in the Introduction to the French Medical System is accurate and current at the time of publication. This book does not claim to contain all information about the medical system in France and other sources or French medical professionals may need to be consulted. The author and the publisher disclaim liability for any misuse or misunderstanding of any information contained herein and for all loss, damage or injury, be it health, financial or otherwise, suffered by any individual or group acting upon or relying on information contained herein. A qualified health practitioner should be consulted in all cases of ill health.

INTRODUCTION TO THE FRENCH MEDICAL SYSTEM

BACKGROUND

The system which provided rapid access to first-class care and surgery had increasingly run into debt by the end of the 1990s through wastage, fraud and abuse, with patients getting second, third and even fourth opinions from GPs and specialists and asking for and obtaining excessive numbers of medicine and pill prescriptions. Visitors from non EEA (European Economic Activity) countries, countries which do not have reciprocal health insurance agreements with France, were assuming identities of friends or family with resident status in France to enjoy health benefits provided by the social security system. And some public and private hospitals and clinics were insisting on costly in-house medical examinations in instances where external medical examination results would have been quite adequate.

Major measures were necessary to reduce the debt while maintaining and even improving the high quality of medical treatment and care received by patients.

1. A 1€ surcharge, which is not reimbursed, to the cost of all visits and consultations.

2. Since 1 January 2006 all residents in France over the age of 16 have been obliged to choose a GP and register their choice, with the GP's signature, at the local national health insurance authority, if they want social security to reimburse the usual proportion of the cost of

visits and consultations. The GP now decides, with certain notable exceptions (see Specialists) if a visit to a specialist is necessary.

3. An increasing number of medicines and pills which are not considered to have any therapeutic effects are reimbursed at a lower rate of 35 per cent by social security or not reimbursed at all. See Pharmacies.

4. Doctors' prescriptions are monitored by government medical inspectors to make sure they are not being too generous.

5. A new plastic health card with identifying photo and a micro chip containing the patient's medical history and data is now being progressively introduced throughout France.

High standards of health care in France will be maintained, with rapid access to preventive and therapeutic care, and choice of doctor, specialist and surgeon still open to patients. Although specialists with particularly good reputations normally have their appointment diaries booked up a few months ahead, waiting lists for hospital surgery are almost unheard of. Visitors and new residents should, however, be aware that, generally, social security reimbursements (unlike in the UK) only cover part of the cost.

Top-up health insurance which is taken out by millions of French people (see Complementary health insurance) should therefore be carefully studied and costed by new residents depending on individual circumstances and medical histories.

Visitors should also note that they will usually have to pay immediately for medical expenses and await reimbursement once the claim they make has been settled through the reciprocal system.

Claims may take months to be paid even using the Internet. Special private holiday insurance cover should therefore be considered.

DOCUMENTS REQUIRED BY VISITORS AND NEW RESIDENTS

Visitors and new residents to France from an EEA country (European Union, Iceland, Liechtenstein, Norway and Switzerland) who wish to be reimbursed as if they were residents in France contributing to the French social security system, have the possibility of obtaining an EHIC card, E106, E109, E112 or E121 entitlement certificates. They should apply for the appropriate form (in the case of the UK from a social security office, post office or on the Internet) well before their visit or move and of course be contributing to the social security system in the country which issues the card or certificate.

EHIC (European Health Insurance Card)

This plastic card, first introduced in June 2004, now completely replaces the former E111 form and is issued free of charge, following a straightforward application. The EHIC card, which is normally valid for one year, now covers all necessary medical treatment following an accident, emergency or illness. The treatment must be effected in a state-run (not a private) establishment and also covers GPs provided the GP is linked to the state health scheme (*conventionné*).

Chronic diseases and pre-existing illnesses are also covered if the person afflicted requires regular treatment during their stay. Special arrangements should be made in advance to ensure facilities are available when and where they are needed.

If pills are taken regularly as a prescribed course of treatment, obtain sufficient pills before departure to cover the visit. Take the prescription with you just in case you lose the pills. If flying out you may also need to show the prescription to airport passenger control.

E112

This certificate covers medical expenses for patients in urgent need of treatment which is unavailable within a reasonable (and painful time) in their country of residence. It is by no means granted automatically. Applicants should already be entitled to the EHIC card. In the UK, an NHS consultant must first send a written recommendation to their patient for treatment outside the UK. The recommendation must subsequently be approved by the local Primary Care Trust (PCT) or Board. All this can take time without any guarantee of approval. The patient may still have to advance money if an E112 is obtained before making a reimbursement claim. In certain instances, however, the PCT may decide to refer the patient to a third-party European medical services provider that works with the NHS under contract, thus getting round the E112 procedure and avoiding any advance payment.

The cost of going as a private patient in France (i.e. outside any reciprocal EEA country agreement) may well be less than in the UK and could be investigated as a last resort.

E109

This is the entitlement certificate required for married couples who decide to set up home in France while the bread-winner continues to work and reside in their original country.

The spouse who resides in France and any accompanying children are immediately covered, provided they register with their E109 on arrival in France at the local state health insurance office, Caisse Primaire d'Assurance Maladie (CPAM). The visiting spouse is covered in the usual way by their EHIC card while the rest of the family under the EEA reciprocal scheme are, in effect, integrated into the French health insurance scheme. The person who is going to remain in the original country of residence makes the application, and in the UK the entitlement certificate is issued by HM Revenue and Customs (Centre for Non-Residents, Room BP1301, Benton Park View, Newcastle upon Tyne, NE98 1ZZ). The application must show all the family members who will be living in France and the CPAM office will confirm and register the family members concerned on the certificate once they are satisfied that identity is proved through passports or other identification papers.

E106 and E121

The E106 certificate is issued for new residents in France who are below the retirement age in their country and will not be working in France. A limited period of health care cover for accidents, illnesses and emergencies, not normally exceeding two years, is allowed. The maximum period will be granted for applicants who have paid all their national insurance contributions throughout their working career and must particularly include fully paid up contributions for the last two income tax years. People who have been self-employed and were not obliged to pay up national insurance contributions should take note. As with the E109 certificate, registration and identification must be made at the local CPAM office. Short Term Incapacity Benefit holders are, however, entitled to cover, as long as their benefit status continues.

If the residents are still below their country's retirement age and not working at the end of the certificate's validity they will, like all adult residents in France, have to pay contributions into the French social security system. Unless free medical cover is granted under the low-income health cover system (see CMU (Couverture Maladie Universelle) below) approximately 8 per cent (in 2006) of income above the CMU threshold figure must be contributed to provide health cover under the state system.

The E121 certificate is issued (in the UK, as with E106, by the Department for Works and Pensions, Newcastle) for new residents who have reached retirement age and are receiving their state pension. For married couples, including common-law marriages, only one of the partners needs to be receiving their state pension for the other partner to be automatically covered. Registration and identification must be made in the usual way with the local CPAM office to provide permanent health care cover for accidents, illnesses and emergencies as long as residence is in France.

Long Term Incapacity Benefit or Severe Disablement Allowance recipients of any age are also entitled to apply for an E121 certificate.

NB: if salaried employment is obtained on arrival in France contributions will automatically be paid to French social security by the employer. Full-time employment – at least 35 hours a week – with an initial qualifying period ensures full state health care benefits, but shorter working weeks may reduce your health benefit entitlements. It is recommended that any proposed part-time employment contract is shown to the CPAM to establish entitlement to health care benefits.

MEDICAL CARE IN EMERGENCIES

Emergency numbers are given at the end of this section.

The SAMU (Service d'Aide Médicale d'Urgence) provides a national network of ambulances always on stand-by, with a doctor (not just a paramedic) and life-support material on board. A doctor is present and deals with the life-threatening situation from the initial phone call to arrival at hospital.

The local fire-brigade (*pompiers*), who double as paramedic ambulance units throughout France, also carry life-support equipment on their vehicles. Nearly 70 per cent of all *pompiers* call-outs are for domestic and road accidents.

REGISTRATION AND HOW THE HEALTH BENEFITS WORK

With the exception of EHIC card holders, all other E certificate holders as described above should register immediately with the local CPAM office not forgetting to give them your French bank account details so that reimbursement payments can be transferred to your account. Consult *sécurité sociale* in the Yellow Pages directory or on the website (www.pagesjaunes.fr) for addresses.

You will be allocated a 13 digit number, *numéro d'immatriculation*, issued by the national statistics department (INSEE) which starts with 1 for men and 2 for women and the year and month of birth. Two additional digits afterwards signify the *département* (Paris, for example is 75) to which the local office is attached. This number appears on the new plastic health card *Carte Vitale II* which is progressively replacing the previous *Carte Vitale* and which is issued to all members of the social security health benefits scheme. The new health card is valid for five years. The *Carte Vitale* (or *Carte Vitale II*) entitles the holder to social security health cover for medical treatment and medicines. Immediate payment, with reimbursement for the portion covered by social security, is made for visits to GPs and specialists.

Ideally, you should choose a GP before you register with the CPAM office, so that you are immediately covered for accidents, emergencies and general medical attention. The declaration form must be signed by both you and the GP. Make sure your GP is linked to the health service (*conventionné*) otherwise you will pay considerably more than the standard 21€ consultation fee (22€ from 1 July, 2007) and will not receive partial reimbursement from the state health scheme. Calling out your GP for a home visit during their usual consultation hours, if you are not well enough to visit the surgery, will of course cost more, as will an 'after-hours' visit from *SOS Médecins* (consult the white phone directory) who operate a 24 hour home visit service.

The choice of GP is important as GPs now decide if visits to specialists for further consultation are necessary. No geographical boundary for registration with a GP is imposed, but near your home, a pharmacist and blood test laboratory, seems sensible. Go along armed with your medical history (you should find this dictionary helpful to translate it!). Check on the surgery door's plate if the GP has a speciality, such as physiotherapy, which is appropriate to your general physical condition. Is the waiting room full or almost empty? Can appointments be made by phone to cut down waiting time? If you do get the initial choice wrong it can always be changed by filling in and getting both signatures on a new declaration form with another GP and then registering it with the CPAM.

NB: if the chosen GP and their locum are absent or unavailable (or in instances of justifiable urgency), and another GP is consulted, reimbursement will be for the normal amount, provided the 'replacement' doctor indicates this when registering your visit. A necessary visit to a GP while absent from home, on holiday or business also falls into this category.

A GP can also be chosen who works in a group practice. If they are not available a colleague in the same practice can be consulted without penalising the reimbursement amount.

Specialists can still however be consulted directly, but the reimbursement amount will be reduced, except for pediatricians, dentists, gynaecologists and oculists who can be contacted directly without penalising reimbursement. There is no requirement to register with any one dentist, gynaecologist or oculist. A patient who has a chronic illness which requires regular care from a specialist can also consult a specialist directly without reimbursement being penalised. Psychiatrists and neuropsychiatrists can also be consulted directly by the 16–25 age group without penalising reimbursement.

Company employees have a pre-contract (and then at least every two years) check-up through the local Service Interprofessionnel de Santé au Travail. This is completely free and takes about 20 minutes. The employees are weighed and measured, have an eye test, a hearing test, a urine test and have their blood pressure taken. Blood-count tests can be requested. GPs should also, on request, give their patients a quick annual check-up. It will not include a urine test or special hearing test and costs slightly more than a standard consultation. Reimbursement for the GP's check-up is on the usual partial basis.

Social security also provides all its members with a completely free comprehensive check-up every five years. This check-up takes upto half a day and checks the heart, blood pressure, hearing, eyesight, teeth, weight, height, vaccinations (checks these are up-to-date and recommends what is required), and a urine test, comprehensive blood test, and colonic/prostrate/breast/lung/cervical cancer tests may be conducted, with immediate X-rays if considered necessary. Ask for it if an invitation is not received after five years.

GPs and specialists can also prescribe X-rays (for suspected bone fractures, diagnosis of osteoporosis (fragile or brittle bones) etc.), physiotherapy treatment, a visit to a chiropodist for necessary false heels or foot support material, orthopaedic material such as compression socks to ease varicose vein problems, etc.

NB: nursing services, physiotherapy and chiropody are reimbursed by social security at 60 per cent, lower than the usual rate (see below) of 70 per cent for medical consultations.

Some doctors and specialists may still be using the *feuille de soins* treatment form. If so ensure that your French social security number (*numéro d'immatriculation*) is on the form and that you date and sign it before sending it off to your CPAM. If you are sending off a form for the first time complete the box for payment (*virement*) account details and enclose a *relevé d'identité bancaire* from your French bank or post office account. Remember when completing forms that the French use a cross on forms instead of a tick. Use of the *Carte Vitale* or *Carte Vitale II* health card through doctors with computer link-up to the *Assurance Maladie* system produces reimbursement in a few days.

CONSULTATION COSTS AND SOCIAL SECURITY HEALTH REIMBURSEMENT PERCENTAGES

Children under the age of 16 do not have to choose a doctor to be reimbursed at the best rate and do not pay the 1€ surcharge for consultations. The set fees (2007) for consulting a GP who is *conventionné* (known as *Secteur 1*) are 26€ for children under two and 24€ for children in the two to six age group. Children in the six to 16 age group pay 21€. All children in these age groups are reimbursed at the rate of 70 per cent. Some GPs who are *conventionnés* are authorised to set higher consultation fees (known as *Secteur 2*), on the grounds that their reputation or additional expertise justifies this, but the reimbursement rate of 70 per cent will still be off the *Secteur 1* fees.

Children in these age groups consulting specialists, such as paediatricians, psychiatrists or heart specialists will pay specialist *Secteur 1* fees – higher than GP *Secteur 1* fees – which differ depending on the speciality. Reimbursement will be at the usual rate of 70 per cent. If a *Secteur 2* specialist is visited, although they charge more, the patient will only receive 70 per cent reimbursement of a set amount which is lower than the *Secteur 1* fee.

Children are entitled to a completely free dental check-up at the ages of six, nine, 12, 15 and 18 provided a *conventionné* dentist of their choice is consulted. The examination must be within three months of their birthday and any treatment required will be reimbursed entirely by social security provided that it is undertaken within six months of the examination. Orthodontic treatment is reimbursed at 100 per cent by social security for children under 16 (no reimbursement over 16) and false teeth are excluded and will be reimbursed at 70 per cent off the social security's scale of prices which are usually not in line with actual dental costs. The local CPAM should send out the check-up invitation when the patient's birthday comes up.

Spectacles for children under six years old are reimbursed at 65 per cent (65 per cent for frames and 65 per cent for glasses) and can be replaced whenever necessary. There are generous allowances for children requiring spectacles in the six to 18 age group.

Patients over 16 are reimbursed on the following basis (2007):
(NB: all reimbursement is minus 1€ surcharge)

GP (patient is registered with)
Secteur 1: 70 per cent of 21€ set fee
Secteur 2: 70 per cent of 21€ *Secteur 1* set fee

GP (patient is not registered with)
Secteur 1: 60 per cent of 21€ set fee
Secteur 2: 60 per cent of 21€ *Secteur 1* set fee

Specialist (with letter from patient's registered GP)
Secteur 1: 70 per cent of 25€ set fee
Secteur 2: 70 per cent of 23€
NB: fees are higher for psychiatrists, neurologists and heart specialists.

Specialist (without letter from patient's registered GP)
Secteur 1: 60 per cent of 25€ (maximum *Secteur 1* specialist fee: 33€)
Secteur 2: 60 per cent of 23€

Neurologist (without letter from patient's registered GP)
Secteur 1: 60 per cent of 37€ (maximum *Secteur 1* neurologist fee: 49€)
Secteur 2: 60 per cent of 34.30€

Heart specialist (without letter from patient's registered GP)
Secteur 1 and *2*: 60 per cent of 45.73€ (maximum *Secteur 1* heart specialist fee: 58€)

NB: all *Secteur 2* specialist fees are not controlled

Gynaecologist and oculist (if patient is registered with GP)
Visit following a course of treatment:
Secteur 1 and *2*: 70 per cent of 28€
Not following a course of treatment:
Secteur 1: 70 per cent of 25€ (maximum fee 32€)
Secteur 2: 60 per cent of 23€ for any visit (no maximum fee)

Gynaecologist and oculist (if patient is not registered with GP)
Secteur 1: 60 per cent of 25€ for any visit (maximum fee 33€)
Secteur 2: 60 per cent of 23€ for any visit (no maximum fee)
NB: people living in the Alsace-Moselle area have a distinct advantage as they are subject to a special health cover regime with a usual reimbursement rate of 90 per cent.

Dental care is reimbursed at the rate of 70 per cent off a scale of prices established by social security; which in practice have little relationship with the actual cost of implants and new ceramic teeth proposed by *Secteur 1* dentists. Extractions and fillings (33.50€ and 16.87€ a tooth respectively in 2007) and scaling are the only work where dentists have to adhere to a set price. Ask for a detailed price (*devis*) before agreeing to any major dental work and discuss the best possible solution.

Patients over 18 requiring spectacles are reimbursed at 65 per cent of a variable tariff for the glass depending on the requirement for correct vision prescribed by the oculist, and also at 65 per cent of a set price (2.84€ in 2007) for frames. The social security's allowance for frames bears little relation to optician's actual prices.

The local CPAM (social security health office) send out reimbursement statements regularly showing what the patient has been reimbursed for and the amount. These statements are set out as follows – with my explanation of the French in brackets. (The example shown is for visits to patient's usual GP and/or specialists with a letter from the patient's usual GP.)

All patients, whether hospitalised or not, receiving medical treatment costing 91€ or more or with a rating of 50 or more, (on a detailed scale established by the Ministry of Health based on complexity and cost of treatment) must pay 18€ towards the cost. This payment is not subject to any social security health reimbursement.

There are however exemptions, notably for: investigative X-rays and associated examinations; transport costs to hospital for treatment costing more than 91€ or with a rating of 50 or more; persons receiving disability pensions; pregnant women (from at least six months into the pregnancy until 12 days after lying-in); hospital fees after the first month as an inpatient, and for employees who fall ill at work or contract illness or disease because of their work. People on low incomes receiving free or financial assistance for medical cover from the government and people living in Alsace-Moselle are also exempt. In all the above cases, all *conventionnés* hospital costs and fees are completely covered (100 per cent) by social security.

Hospitalisation, emergencies apart, is arranged by the GP or specialist. The patient can choose their hospital or clinic. Although there is no

Dates	Nature des prestations (treatment received)	Montant payé (amount paid)	Base du remboursement (amount taken into account for refund calculation)	Taux (rate)	Montant versé (amount refunded)
Parcours coordonné Médecin traitant Généraliste Secteur 1 (visit to usual GP who is registered Secteur 1)	xxx	xxx	70%	xxx	
Participation forfaitaire (surcharge contribution)				- 1,00 €	
Parcours coordonné Médecin correspondant (Appropriate specialist with letter from usual GP) Acte tech, médical Secteur 2 (Specific medical treatment Secteur 2)	xxx	xxx	70%	xxx	
Participation forfaitaire (surcharge contribution)				- 1,00 €	

marked difference between the quality of care available in public and private clinics and hospitals, the scope of care and medical equipment available is usually wider in a public hospital. As regards reimbursement, ideally choose a public hospital.

Admission should be accompanied by presentation of the plastic *Vitale* health card (or EHIC card if you are a visitor), the GP's letter and any appropriate medical records – X-rays, blood test results, vaccinations card and in the case of an accident at work, a declaration form completed by the employer. A complementary health insurance certificate or holiday insurance certificate should also be registered by the admissions department.

The basic cost (2007) for meals and a bed is 16€ a day in hospitals and clinics, and 12€ a day in special psychiatric units. The *forfait hospitalier* is not covered by social security. The following are, however, exempt: patients suffering from employment-associated accidents and illnesses, pregnant women (over five months pregnant until 12 days after lying-in), parents whose newborn child has been hospitalised until upto 30 days after birth, patients receiving after care at home, people living in Alsace-Moselle, parents whose under 20 handicapped child lives in a specialised establishment, patients benefiting from a military pension and state-assisted low income groups.

The cost of a single room and the higher (*dépassement d'honoraire*) cost of any authorised *Secteur 2* doctors' fees are not reimbursed by social security. However, the cost of a single room which is necessary on prescribed medical grounds will be reimbursed.

Public hospitals should all be able to use the plastic health cards for registration and reimbursement purposes, although only about 10 per cent of them (2007) have all their previous patients' medical history on computer. Once the hospitals/clinics admission certificate has been completed send it off to the local CPAM.

Hospitalisation fees are covered at the rate of 80 per cent by social security and the balance amount, the *ticket modérateur*, must be paid when leaving the hospital or clinic. Complementary health insurance and social security cover can together provide 100 per cent medical and surgical cover and a *tiers payant* clause in the complementary policy automatically pays the *ticket modérateur* so no money has to be advanced. If you have been admitted to a *nonconventionnée* private clinic, all fees must be paid when you leave, with reimbursement from social security and any complementary health cover. Check before admission on *hors convention* prices and exactly how much will be reimbursed by social security and complementary insurance.

Complementary health insurance is strongly recommended to complete the cover provided by social security. Mutual benefit societies (*mutuelles*) – consult *mutuelles* in the Yellow Pages or on www.pagesjaunes.fr – and banks provide this.

NB: there is usually an initial probationary period of three months for first-time subscribers during which no claims can be made. Existing policy holders who decide to change their complementary insurance provider – perhaps tempted by a no-premium offer for the first three months – can, however, usually make any claims, and be reimbursed immediately.

In comparing policies, basic cover, i.e. with the lowest premium payments, should offer, with social security benefits, the following:

- 100 per cent cover for all medical and surgical hospital costs and fees including ambulance cost, but exclude a single room.

NB: with the exception of emergencies, a doctor's letter should always be obtained before transportation, prescribing whether ambulance, taxi, private car or public transport is appropriate. For regular journeys of over 50 km, individual journeys of over 150 km one-way, and airline flights and maritime transport, submit a doctor's letter to the local CPAM for prior authorisation. The usual social security reimbursement rate is 65 per cent with 100 per cent social security reimbursement for residents in Alsace-Moselle;

• 100 per cent cover for at least 60 days to cover hospital costs and fees in a hospital offering specialised treatment, but exclude a single room;

• 100 per cent cover for all consultations (visits to GPs and specialists); general medical and specialist treatment; speech and physical therapy and nursing care; X-rays, scans, etc. and blood tests;

• 100 per cent cover for those medicines and pills (see Pharmacies) which are partially reimbursed by social security;

• 100 per cent cover for dental extractions and fillings, and an annual limited amount for certain types of false teeth classed as prostheses, which excludes implants;

• 100 per cent cover for prostheses for the disabled and a (small) limited annual amount for hearing aids.

Social security cover apart, complementary insurance should offer:

• A limited annual amount towards the cost of prescribed spa bath treatment.

• A small contribution towards the cost of spectacles including the frames.

Some organisations also offer price reductions on leisure-time activities, e.g. cinema tickets, holidays and sports. Policy premiums vary according to age at entry, but are considerably less than private plan health cover premiums in the UK. Subscribe to a policy with a *tiers payant* direct payment clause to avoid personally advancing payment.

LOW-INCOME HEALTH COVER

Foreign families (from within the EEA or Switzerland) with at least three months continuous residence in France and annual household income which was below 7083€ in 2005 do not have to make any social security contributions to be covered for full state health care benefits, Couverture Maladie Universelle (CMU). Reimbursement is made in the usual way as if they were contributing to the system.

If the joint income of a couple did not exceed 897.35€ monthly (2006/7 year) they qualify, for a year, for the CMU *complémentaire* system health cover, free of charge and free of advance payments, for hospital fees such as the daily subsistence cost (*forfait hospitalier*), and for *dépassement d'honoraire* costs and fees, particularly for dental care, hearing aids and spectacles.

Another possible case is *l'aide complémentaire santé* which applies to incomes not exceeding the CMU *complémentaire* qualifying income thresholds by more than 20 per cent (for the year 2007). There is a sliding scale of financial assistance, culminating in 400€ a year for the over 60s, as a contribution to the cost of complementary health insurance policy premiums. The contribution cannot exceed the premium amount.

Qualifying income figures change annually, although they usually remain unchanged during the year, for these low-income aids. Verify them with the local CPAM, and ask for a qualifying certificate if proven income falls into any of the above categories.

PHARMACIES

Many pharmacies are no longer open on Saturday afternoons since the 35 hour working week was introduced. They do however shut late during the week, and will usually close for lunch. All pharmacies which are open have a flashing neon cross sign prominently fixed outside their premises. There is always at least one pharmacy open after hours or on Sundays to serve the local community. Look for the *Pharmacie de garde* or *Pharma garde* details in the *Infos Services* or *Infos pratiques* announcements in local newspapers.

An increasing number of medicines and pills are not reimbursed by social security, even if they are prescribed by doctors and it may pay to shop around as pharmacy retail prices are not fixed and can vary considerably. If you are going to be prescribed a *médicament* regularly, ask your doctor if it is still on the reimbursement, or partial reimbursement, list.

Reimbursement of pills and medicines accounts for around one third of all health care reimbursement costs in France, about twice the total amount reimbursed for dental, eyes and auditive care. The French are still by far the champion pill takers in Europe, although, since 1999, literally hundreds of pills and medicines have been downgraded for reimbursement rate or are no longer reimbursed at all. For example, in March 2006, the Ministry of Health classed over 150 *médicaments* ineffective and no longer reimbursable, and a month earlier a decision was taken to progressively phase out reimbursement for all pills or medicine for treatment of varicose veins (*veinotoniques*) as their effectiveness – compared to surgery or wearing compression socks – is in doubt. (*Veinotoniques* or their equivalents are almost unknown in the UK).

Heart pills and insulin are essential medicines and reimbursed by social security at 100 per cent.

Major or important medicines (with a white label on their packaging) are reimbursed at 65 per cent; moderate or 'weak'medicines providing comfort rather than cure (with a blue label on their packaging) are reimbursed at 35 per cent, and the *veinotoniques* are at present subject to a special reduced reimbursement rate of 15 per cent. They will come off the reimbursement list in 2008.

NB: not all *mutuelles* compensate, with a higher rate of complementary reimbursement, for these reductions.

The reduction in reimbursement rates for medicines and pills operates alongside a continuous campaign, initiated by social security through pharmacies, which proposes people buy identical molecule products – generic products – which are cheaper than the brand on the doctor's prescription. There is no obligation to accept a generic product, although their consumption helps to reduce the health system's debt.

Register with a local pharmacy with the *Carte Vitale* and up-to-date complementary health insurance policy details with a *tiers payant* clause and no advance payment will be made for the reimbursement elements. Note, however that the health insurance administration offices in some *départements* now penalise patients who will not accept a generic product by withdrawing the *tiers payant* facility from their reimbursement procedure. This means that patients now have to pay immediately for the total cost of prescription products with reimbursement from both social security and complementary health insurance following.

Pharmacists also sell body creams, hair care products, toothpaste, toothbrushes and baby products which are of better quality, and more expensive, than those sold in supermarkets. Energy drinks and sweets that are not sold in supermarkets are also available. Small orthopaedic items such as back support belts and arm slings are sold or may be supplied on prescription by pharmacists.

BLOOD TESTS

GPs also prescribe blood tests for sugar/cholesterol/acidity etc. and blood counts which should be reimbursed completely, or require no advance payment with a good basic complementary health insurance policy containing a *tiers payant* clause. Register as for a pharmacy. Many tests require empty stomachs so the *laboratoire d'analyses médicales* will take blood samples early morning, before breakfast. Check beforehand with the GP if an empty stomach (*à jeun*) is required.

Strictly speaking the GP should be consulted afterwards to run through the test results with the patient, although qualified staff who are supervised by the biologist doctor who runs the blood test laboratory should alert the patient of any 'bad' results. Ask if the results are satisfactory or not if no information is volunteered.

VACCINATIONS

The following vaccinations are reimbursed by social security (certain conditions apply): diphtheria, German measles, haemophilia, varicella, hepatitis B, measles, mumps, poliomyelitis, (anti)tetanus, tuberculosis, whooping cough, pneumococcus diseases; and flu for the over 65s.

Doctors should be consulted for obligatory and recommended vaccinations for babies and young children. The BCG (anti-tuberculosis) vaccination is still obligatory for all children over six before they can go to school or to any other child education/childcare centre such as kindergartens and playgroups. Diphtheria, tetanus and poliomyelitis vaccinations are recommended for adults every ten years. Hepatitis A vaccination is recommended for people working with children or food, for those working in waste-water processing, for those working in the health profession and for homosexual men. Vets and their assistants, pound employees, gamekeepers and abattoir personnel are recommended to have (anti) rabies injections and all doctors, depending on the precise nature of their work, must be inoculated against diphtheria, poliomyelitis, hepatitis B, typhoid, TB and whooping cough.

EMERGENCY NUMBERS

SAMU (Service d'Aide Médicale d'Urgence): 15
Local fire brigade and resuscitation assistance (*pompiers*): 18
From a mobile phone: 112

Some English-language websites

www.bestfrancemagazine.co.uk
www.exclusivehealthcare.com
www.expathealthdirect.co.uk
www.know-insurance.co.uk
www.soficas.fr

NOTES

TERMINOLOGIE ADMINISTRATIVE, CLINIQUES, HOPITAUX ET CABINETS PARAMEDICAUX

ADMINISTRATIVE TERMS, CLINICS, HOSPITALS AND PARAMEDICAL ESTABLISHMENTS

The French masculine *m* or feminine *f* gender is given immediately after each noun.

acte *m* médical medical procedure

acte *m* de naissance birth certificate

acte *m* de décès death certificate

âge moyen *adj* middle age

agréé(e) *adj* officially approved, registered

allocation *f* personnalisée à l'autonomie (APA) home help (subsidised) for the over 60s requiring physical assistance

allocation *f* de maternité maternity benefit

ambulance *f* municipale town ambulance service

analyses *fpl* medical test/investigation

arrêté *m* municipal municipal by-law (e.g. to forbid sea bathing in polluted water)

Assistance Publique (AP) *f* public general hospital

assurance *f* maladie health insurance

assurance *f* maladie complémentaire complementary health insurance

assurance *f* indemnité journalière income accident/sickness cover

assurance en cas d'invalidité *f* permanente totale permanent total disablement insurance usually providing lump sum payment

assurance *f* vie whole-life insurance with savings plan

assurance *f* décès death insurance (allows your family to claim a pre-agreed amount after your death)

attestation *f* médicale doctor's certificate

bilan *m* de santé health check-up report

cabinet *m* de consultation consulting room

cabinet *m* médical surgery

cabinet *m* de kinésithérapie/ de rééducation fonctionelle physiotherapist's surgery

cabinet *m* de médecine générale GP practice

cabinet *m* de pédicure-podologue chiropodist's surgery

cabinet *m* de rééducation fonctionnelle physiotherapist's surgery

Caisse d'Allocations Familiales (CAF) *f* family allowance office

Caisse Primaire d'Assurance Maladie (CPAM) *f* state health insurance office

campagne *f* anti-tabac anti-smoking campaign

carnet *m* de santé medical record

carnet *m* de vaccination vaccination record

carnet *m* de maternité maternity record book

carte *f* à puce plastic card with electronic chip

carte *f* d'invalidité civile disability card

Carte Vitale *f* plastic health card

Carte Vitale *f* II new generation plastic health card

centre *m* anti-poison poisons unit

centre *m* de balnéothérapie balneotherapy centre

centre *m* de cancérologie, centre anti-cancéreux cancer hospital

centre *m* de convalescence convalescent home

centre *m* de dépistage medical testing centre

centre *m* de dyalyse kidney dialysis unit

centre *m* hospitalier général general hospital

Centre *m* Hospitalier Régional/Intercommunal (CHR/CHI) regional/ community hospital

Centre *m* Hospitalier Universitaire (CHU) teaching or university hospital

centre *m* de planning familial family planning clinic

certificat *m* de consolidation doctor's certificate indicating that patient's condition is stable, following work accident/illness

centre *m* médico-social outpatient health care centre
centre *m*/unité *f* de moyen séjour medium-stay hospital
centre/poste *m* de secours first-aid centre/post
centre *m* de quarantaine isolation hospital
centre de santé *m* health care centre
centre *m*/unité *f* de long séjour long-term treatment hospital
certificat *m* médical medical certificate
certificat *m* de décès doctor's death certificate
certificat *m* de vaccination vaccination certificate
chef *m* de service head of medical department, consultant
chef *m* de clinique registrar
Classification *f* Commune des Actes Médicaux (CCAM) official list of medical treatments, tests and investigations
clinique *f* hospital service which teaches a medical speciality **or** private medical, surgical or psychiatric establishment
clinique *f* d'accouchement maternity hospital
clinique *f* dentaire dental clinic
clinique *f* chirurgicale surgical clinic
clinique-polyclinique *f* private general hospital
clinique *f* prénatale prenatal clinic
clinique *f* psychiatrique psychiatric clinic
codage *m* des actes system used by social security to register their reimbursements
commissariat *m* de police national police station
congé *m* maladie sick leave
consultation *f* GP or specialist surgery visit
consultation *f* generaliste GP surgery
consultation *f* libre GP surgery visit without appointment
conventionné *adj* approved status for social security, linked to the state health service
cordon *m* sanitaire quarantine line

corps *m* médical the medical profession

décharge *f* de responsabilité hospital discharge form

déclaration *f* d'accident du travail work accident report form

délivrer *v* to give/issue (a prescription), to dispense (medicine)

demande *f* d'entente préalable approval request for reimbursement (for certain treatments)

dépassement *m* exceptionnel higher than standard fees charged by approved specialists

dépassement *m* permanent higher than standard fees charged by approved specialists for any treatment, because they have special expertise

dossier *m* médical medical records

droit *m* médical medical law

d'âge moyen *adj* middle-aged

examen *m* clinique complet medical check-up

externe *m/f* des hôpitaux medical student in fourth to sixth year

feuille *f* de soins treatment form (for reimbursements)

forfait *m* journalier set daily subsistence fee due to hospitals

frais *mpl* costs; fees

frais *mpl* réels actual expenditure

honoraires *mpl* de médecin doctor's fee

honoraires *mpl* libres fees higher than the *conventionnés* fees approved by social security

honoraires *mpl* médicaux medical fees

hôpital *m* hospital

hôpital *m* conventionné private/public hospital linked to social security system for direct payment or full-rate reimbursement

hôpital *m* nonconventionné private hospital/clinic outside social security link-up, possibly with partial reimbursement status

hôpital *m* de court séjour short-stay hospital

hôpital *m* pour enfants children's hospital

hôpital *m* de jour outpatients department

hôpital *m* psychiatrique psychiatric hospital

hospitalisation *f* à domicile (HAD) supervised home convalescence

indice *m* de pollution atmosphérique air quality index

interdiction *f* absolue/ formelle de fumer strictly no smoking (NB. No smoking is in force in all enclosed public areas and on means of transport. By 2008 all private businesses, including bars, must provide a separate, enclosed area with extractor fans for smokers).

interne *m/f* des hôpitaux house officer, houseman (responsible to head of department)

interne *m/f* en médecine house physician

interne *m/f* en chirurgie house surgeon

intervention *f* chirurgicale; opération *f* medical operation

livret *m* d'accueil hospital information booklet

magasin *m* de produits diététiques health food shop

maison *f* de retraite retirement home

maître nageur *m* -euse *f*; sauveteur *m* -euse *f* (MNS) lifeguard

majeur *attrib* aged over 18

maternité *f* maternity clinic (in a hospital)

médecin *m* reférent GP linked to health scheme following the changes which were announced in 1998

médecin *m* traitant patient's chosen doctor (for social security reimbursement purposes)

médicaments *mpl* de confort pain relief medication

médicament *m* sans ordonnance non-prescription/over-the-counter medicine

membre *m* d'une association de gestion agréée member of association of administration services organisations (member doctors print this on their prescription forms)

mutuelle *f* mutual benefit society

norme *f* française (NF) label on goods and services for approved French standards of quality, safety and suitability

nonconventionné(e) *adj* not linked to the social security system

numéro *m* d'immatriculation social security number

Organisation *f* Mondiale de la Santé (OMS) World Health Organisation (WHO)

ordonnance *f* prescription

uniquement sur ordonnance only on prescription

Ordre *m* des Médecins France's medical register

poste *m* de secours first-aid post

prestations *fpl* en espèces cash payment benefits

prestations *fpl* en nature benefits (e.g. transport to and from a hospital)

prise en charge *f* totale costs reimbursed entirely by social security

professions *fpl* de santé health care professions

protocole *m* thérapeutique medical protocol

quatrième âge *m* over 75 age group

régime *m* commun social security hospitalisation scheme

régime *m* d'assurance maladie health insurance scheme

régime *m* de la sécurité sociale social security system

régime *m* des hôpitaux hospital system/regulations

relevé *m* d'identité bancaire (RIB) document with personal bank account particulars

résidence *f* médicalisée nursing home

santé *f* publique public health
sécurité *f* sociale social security
service *f* de consultation externe outpatients department
services *mpl* de santé health services
système *m* de santé health system
Secteur 1 *m* doctors/specialists who apply the social security's chart for fees (see *tarif de convention*)
Secteur 2 *m* doctors/specialists who are authorised to apply higher fees than the social security's chart for fees (see *tarif de convention*)
service *m* hospitalier de consultation externe outpatient's clinic
soins *mpl* dentaires dental care
soins *mpl* infirmiers nursing care
tarif *m* de convention (TC) standard-rate hospital and doctors' fees from which social security apply their reimbursement percentages
tarif *m* de responsabilité (TR) social security price chart (particularly for medicines) from which social security apply their reimbursement percentages
tiers payant *m* direct payment by insurers
ticket *m* modérateur (TM) patient's contribution (can be covered by complementary health insurance)
troisième âge *m* retirement years

virement *m* bancaire bank transfer
visite *f* call-out visit

NOTES

ADMINISTRATIVE TERMS, CLINICS, HOSPITALS AND PARAMEDICAL ESTABLISMENTS

TERMINOLOGIE ADMINISTRATIVE, CLINIQUES, HOPITAUX ET CABINETS PARAMEDICAUX

Any comments or further explanations are in brackets after the English.

The French masculine *m* or feminine *f* gender is given immediately after each translated noun.

actual expenditure frais *mpl* réels

approval request for reimbursement (for certain treatment) demande d'entente préalable *f*

approved social security status for higher than standard-rate fees conventionné avec honoraires *mpl* libres

approved status for social security conventionné *adj*

balneotherapy centre centre *m* de balnéothérapie

bank account, document with personal particulars relevé *m* d'identité bancaire (RIB)

bank transfer virement *m* bancaire

benefits (e.g. transport to and from a hospital) prestations *fpl* en nature

birth certificate acte *m* de naissance

call-out visit visite *f*

cancer hospital centre *m* de cancérologie; centre d'oncologie; centre anti-cancéreux

chiropodist's surgery cabinet *m* de pédicure-podologie

combined pharmacy-parapharmaceutical outlet pharmacie-parapharmacie *f*

contribution from patient (usually covered by complementary health insurance) ticket *m* modérateur (TM)

costs reimbursed entirely by social security prise en charge *f* totale

costs; fees frais *mpl*

death certificate acte *m* de décès
dental care soins *mpl* dentaires
dental clinic clinique *f* dentaire
direct payment by insurers tiers payant *m*
disability card carte *f* d'invalidité civile
doctor's certificate attestation *f* médicale
doctor, patient's chosen (for social security reimbursement purposes) médecin *m* traitant

elderly (post middle age to 75) troisième âge *m* **(over 75)** quatrième âge *m*

family allowance office Caisse d'Allocations familiales (CAF) *f*
family planning clinic centre *m* de planning familial

general hospital centre *m* hospitalier général
GP surgery consultation *f* généraliste
GP surgery visit without appointment consultation *f* libre

health card Carte Vitale *f*
health card (new generation) Carte Vitale II *f*
health check-up report bilan *m* de santé
health food shop magasin *m* de produits diététiques
higher than standard fees from approved specialists dépassement *m* permanent
higher than standard fees charged by approved specialists dépassement *m* exceptionnel
home help (subsidised) for the over 60s requiring physical assistance allocation *f* personnalisée à l'autonomie (APA)
hospital hôpital *m*
hospital information booklet livret *m* d'accueil
hospital discharge form décharge *f* de responsabilité

kidney dialysis unit centre *m* de dyalyse

long-term treatment hospital centre *m*/unité *f* de long séjour

maternity benefit allocation *f* de maternité
maternity hospital/clinic clinique *f* d'accouchement, **(in a hospital)** maternité *f*
maternity record book carnet *m* de maternité
medical certificate certificat *m* de santé
medical records dossier *m* médical
medical protocol protocole *m* thérapeutique
medical testing centre centre *m* de dépistage
medical procedure acte *m* médical
medium-stay hospital centre *m*/unité *f* de moyen séjour
mutual benefit society mutuelle *f*

nursing care soins *mpl* infirmiers

outpatients department hôpital *m* de jour; services *mpl* de consultation externe
outpatient health care centre centre *m* médicosocial
over 75 age group quatrième âge *m*

pain-relief medication médicament *m* de confort
physiotherapist's surgery cabinet *m* de kinésithérapie/de rééducation fonctionnelle
plastic card with electronic chip carte *f* à puce
police station, national commissariat *m* de police
prescription ordonnance *f*
private general hospital clinique-polyclinique *f*
private/public hospital linked to social security for direct payment or full-rate reimbursement
hôpital *m* conventionné
private hospital/clinic outside social security link, possibly with partial reimbursement status hôpital *m* nonconventionné

psychiatric clinic clinique *f* psychiatrique
psychiatric hospital hôpital *m* psychiatrique
public assistance service assistance *f* publique
public general hospital Assistance Publique (AP) *f*

regional/community hospital Centre *m* Hospitalier Régional/ Intercommunal (CHR/CHI)
retirement home maison *f* de retraite

short-stay hospital hôpital *m* de court séjour
social security sécurité *f* sociale
social security hospitalisation scheme régime *m* commun
social security price chart from which reimbursement percentages are calculated tarif *m* de responsabilité (TR)
social security system, linked to conventionné *adj*
social security system, not linked to nonconventionné *adj*
standard-rate hospital and doctors' fees from which social security reimbursement percentages are calculated tarif *m* de convention (TC)
state health insurance office Caisse Primaire d'Assurance Maladie (CPAM) *f*
subsistence fee (daily) due to hospitals forfait *m* journalier
supervised home convalescence hospitalisation *f* à domicile (HAD)
surgery visit (GP or specialist) consultation *f*
surgical clinic clinique *f* chirurgicale

teaching or university hospital Centre *m* Hospitalier Universitaire (CHU)
treatment form (for reimbursements) feuille *f* de soins
town ambulance service ambulance *f* municipale

NOTES

TERMES MEDICAUX, DE SANTE ET DE PHARMACIE, PRODUITS ET PLANTES

MEDICAL, HEALTH AND PHARMACY TERMS, PRODUCTS AND PLANTS

Comments and brief explanations, where considered appropriate, are in brackets after the translation.

The French masculine *m* or feminine *f* gender is given immediately after each noun.

à ut. av. (abbrev = à utiliser avant) use before (date on medicines)
abasie *f* abasia (inability to walk)
abcès *m* abscess
abcès *m* gingival gumboil abscess
abdomen *m* abdomen; stomach
abdomen *m* sans préparation abdominal X-ray without prior treatment
douleur *f* abdominale abdominal pain
abdominaux *mpl* abdominal muscles
étage *m* abdomino-pelvien abdominal and lower abdominal area
abducteur *m* abductor muscle
abduction *f* abduction
abduction *f* active patient spreads limb away from their body
abduction *f* forcée doctor applies pressure, forcing limb away from patient's body
abduction *f* passive doctor spreads patient's limb away from body
aberration *f* aberration (abnormal)
aberration *f* chromosomique chromosomal aberration
ablation *f* surgical operation to remove organ or tumor
abord *m* initial incision area in surgical operation **or** beginning of a course of treatment
aboulie *f* ab(o)ulia (mental disorder with loss of willpower)
aboulique *f* person suffering from ab(o)ulia
abrasion *f* surgical smoothening of the skin **or** natural wearing down of body parts

absence ***f*** **de mémoire** temporary mental blank

absorption ***f*** absorption

accès ***m*** sudden burst/bout/fit/attack

accès ***m*** **de fièvre** bout of fever

accès ***m*** **de toux** bout of coughing

accident ***f*** **cardiaque** heart attack

accident ***m*** **vasculaire cérébral** stroke

accident ***m*** **ischémique (cérébral) transitoire** stroke which lasts less than 24 hours

accolement ***m*** organs (normally) immediately adjacent

accommodation ***f*** accommodation (automatic focussing function of the eyes)

accouchement ***m*** childbirth/delivery

accouchement ***m*** **à terme** full-term delivery

accouchement ***m*** **avant terme** early birth

accouchement ***m*** **par le siège** breech birth

accouchement ***m*** **prématuré** premature birth

accouchement ***m*** **provoqué** induced delivery

accouchement ***m*** **spontané** easy childbirth (minimum medical assistance)

accoucheur -euse ***m/f*** obstetrician

accoutumance ***f*** increasing dependence on medicine or pill

accroître ***v*** **son capital santé** to build up one's health

accumulation ***f*** accumulation, for example of fatty deposits

achalasie ***f*** abnormal closing up of the gullet or intestines

acharnement ***m*** **thérapeutique** uncomfortable prolongation of life by medical intervention

achondroplasie ***f*** achondroplasia (hereditary bone growth reduction)

acide ***m*** **acétylsalicylique/aspirine** ***f*** aspirin

acide ***m*** **ascorbique/vitamine C** ***f*** ascorbic acid (Vitamin C)

acide ***m*** **citrique** citric acid

acide ***m*** **folique** folic acid

acide *m* ribonucléique ribonucleic acid (controls the body's protein composition)

acide *m* urique uric acid

acidité *f* gastrique gastric acidity

acidocétose *f* increased blood acidity (a complication in serious diabetes cases)

acidose *f* acidosis (blood with high acidity)

acné *f* juvénile childhood/adolescence acne

acné *f* rosacée acne rosacea (swollen, visible blood vessels)

acoumétrie *f* acoumetry (hearing evaluation)

acouphène *m* tinnitus (ringing in ears)

acrocyanose *f* poor blood circulation (causing 'bluish' fingers/toes)

acromégalie *f* acromegaly (growth hormone disorder causing gigantism)

acromion *m* section of spatula joining arm to chest

acroparesthésie *f* pins and needles sensation (prolongation can be result of a tumour or rheumatism)

acuité *f* acuteness; sensitivity

acupuncture *f* acupuncture

addictologue *m* addiction specialist

adducteur *m* adductor muscle

adduction *f* adduction (action of closing limbs to body)

adénite *f* adenitis (swelling of lymph nodes)

adénocarcinome *m* a cancerous tumour or growth

adénofibrome *m* benign growth (often on breast)

adénoïdectomie *f* surgical removal of adenoids

adénome *m* benign tumour/growth

adénopathie *f* general term for ganglion disorders

adhérence *f* abnormal adhesion of two body parts

adhérence *f* préputiale abnormal foreskin covering (in young boy)

adiposité *f* adiposity (excess body fat)

adjuvant *m* adjuvant, complements treatment but

not effective if used as sole treatment

adoucissant ***m*** skin softener lotion

adrénaline ***f*** adrenalin

aérocolie ***f*** aerocoly (excessive air in the large intestine)

aéroiléie ***f*** (excessive air in the small intestine)

aérogastrie ***f*** aerogastria (excessive air in the stomach)

aérophagie ***f*** aerophagy (temporary excess amount of air in the stomach, often after a meal)

affection ***f*** ailment, affection

âge ***m*** **mental** mental age (based on results of IQ tests)

âge ***m*** **osseux** bone development time graph compared to child's real age

âgées, personnes ***fpl*** the elderly

agent ***m*** **coagulant du sang** blood clotting agent

agent ***m*** **thérapeutique** therapeutic medicine

agglutination ***f*** agglutination (clumping of bacteria, etc.)

agglutinine ***f*** agglutinin (antibody etc. causing clumping)

agglutinines ***fpl*** **irrégulières** rare collection of substances in the blood that should be identified before any blood transfusion

agoraphobie ***f*** agoraphobia

agrafe ***f*** surgical clip

agranulocytose ***f*** abnormal reduction in white corpuscles

aide-soignant(e) ***m/f*****,** nurse's aide

aigreurs ***fpl*****/brûlures** ***fpl*** **(d'estomac)** heartburn

aigu(ë) ***adj*** acute; sharp

aiguille ***f*** needle

aiguille ***f*** **pour piqûres** hypodermic needle

ail ***m*** garlic

aine ***f*** groin

aire ***f*** **pulmonaire** lung X-ray

aisselle ***f*** armpit

AIT (see accident ischémique (cérébral) transitoire)

alaise ***f*** drawsheet

alaise ***f*** **jetable** single-use drawsheet

alèze ***f*** drawsheet

alcoolique *m* dependant alcoholic
appareil de massage pour les pieds *m* foot massaging apparatus
appui-dos *m* backrest
albinisme *m* albinism
albumine *f* albumin (protein in egg-white, blood, milk)
(hypo-)albuminémie *f* insufficient protein content in the blood
(hyper-)albuminémie *f* excessive protein content in the blood
albuminurie *f* albuminuria (abnormal protein count in the urine)
alcaloïde *m* alkaloid
alcool *m* à 90 surgical spirits
alcool *m* éthylique absolu pure ethyl alcohol
alcoolémie *f* amount of alcohol in the blood
Alcooliques Anonymes *mpl* Alcoholics Anonymous
alcoolisé(e) *adj* containing alcohol
très peu alcoolisé(e) *adj* very low alcohol content
alcoolisme *m* alcoholism
alcoologue *m* specialist in medical treatment for alcoholism
alcootest *m* Breathalyser®
faire subir *v* un alcootest to breathalyse
algie *f* algia; pain
-algie -algia (at end of words) denoting pain
algie *f* vasculaire de la face unexplained condition with bouts of violent headaches
algodystrophie *f* sympathique disorder of the joints
algues *fpl* algae; seaweed
(aux) algues *fpl* laminaires product containing seaweed (used in thalassotherapy)
aliments *mpl* de régime diet foods
alitement *m* confinement to bed
allaitement *m* au biberon bottle feeding
allaitement *m* maternel breast-feeding
allaitement *m* mixte breast and bottle feeding
allaiter *v* to (breast) feed

allaiter ***v*** **au biberon** to bottle feed
allégation ***f*** a doctor's written report of what a patient says
allergène ***m*** allergen
allergie ***f*** allergy
allergie ***f*** **cutanée** skin allergy
allergie ***f*** **de contact** contact allergy
allergie ***f*** **respiratoire** respiratory allergy
allergique ***adj*** allergic
allergologie ***f*** study of allergies
allopathie ***f*** allopathy (conventional therapeutic method of treatment)
alopécie ***f*** alopecia (temporary, partial or complete hair loss)
alphabloquant ***m*** alpha-blocker
alvéole ***f*** **pulmonaire** alveolus (oxygen passage to the blood, in the lungs)
alvéole ***f*** **dentaire** tooth socket
alvéolite ***f*** inflammation of the lungs
Alzheimer ***f*****, maladie d'** Alzheimer's disease
altérer ***v*** to deteriorate
amalgame ***m*** **dentaire** dental amalgam
ambulance ***f*** ambulance
aménorrhée ***f*** **primaire** complete absence of menstruation in an adolescent girl
aménorrhée ***f*** **secondaire** occasional menstruation absences in a patient who otherwise menstruates normally
amiante ***f*****; asbeste** ***m*** asbestos
amibe ***f*** amoeba; ameba (tropical parasite)
amibiase ***f*** tropical infection by amoeba
amincissant(e) ***adj*** slimming (product, etc.)
a minima ***adj*** hairline (of fracture)
ammoniac ***m*** ammonia (gas)
ammoniaque ***f*** ammonia (liquid)
amnésie ***f*** amnesia
amnésie ***f*** **antérograde** amnesia following a stroke or brain condition
amniocentèse ***f*** amniocentesis (amniotic fluid removal from the womb of pregnant mothers)

amnios ***m*** amnion (innermost membrane enclosing the embryo)

amniotique ***adj*** amniotic (of innermost membrane)

liquide ***m*** **amniotique** amniotic fluid

(en) amont ***m*** the 'up' side of artery (to stem bleeding)

amphétamine ***f*** amphetamine (stimulant)

ampliation ***f*** **thoracique** breathing exercise which swells chest

ampoule ***f*** blister; phial; ampulla

ampoule ***f*** **rectale** rectal ampulla

couvert(e) ***adj*** **d'ampoules** full of blisters

amputation ***f*** amputation

amygdalectomie ***f*** tonsillectomy (surgical removal of tonsils)

amygdales ***fpl*** tonsils

amygdalite ***f*** tonsillitis

amyotrophie ***f*** muscle wasting condition

anabolisant ***m*** anabolic steroid

anal(e) ***adj*** anal

analgésie ***f*** analgesia (absence/relief of pain)

analgésique ***m*** **and** ***adj*** analgesic; painkiller

anaphylaxie ***f*** extreme, possibly life-threatening reaction to an antigen

choc ***m*** **anaphylactique** anaphylactic shock

analyse ***f*** **de sang** blood test

analyse ***f*** **d'urine** urine test

anasarque ***f*** anasarca or dropsy (excess of fluid in body tissues or cavities)

anastomose ***f*** bypass operation (heart, alimentary canal, etc.)

androgène ***m*** androgen (male hormone)

androgyne ***m/f/adj*** androgyne

andropause ***f*** male menopause

anéchogène ***adj*** imperceptible with an ultrasound scan

anémie ***f*** anaemia

hypochromique ***adj*** reduction in number of red corpuscles

hyposidérémique ***adj*** reduction in number of red corpuscles and iron deficiency in the blood

pernicieuse progressive ***adj*** pernicious anaemia

anesthésie ***f*** anaesthesia; loss of body part sensitivity

anesthésie générale ***f*** general anaesthesia

anesthésie locale ***f*** local anaesthesia

anesthésie péridurale ***f*** epidural anaesthesia (into lower area of spinal cord)

anesthésique ***m and adj*** anaesthetic

anesthésiste ***m/f*** anaesthetist

anévrisme ***m;*** **anévrysme** ***m*** aneurism; aneurysm (abnormal swelling of artery)

rupture ***f*** **d'anévri(y)sme** aneurysmal rupture (life-threatening)

angéite ***f*** blood-system vascular disease

angélique ***f*** angelica plant

angine ***f*** throat infection; tonsillitis

angine ***f*** **blanche** whitish infection in the throat

angine ***f*** **pharyngienne** infection at the back and bottom of the throat

angine ***f*** **rouge** tonsillitis

angine ***f*** **virale** viral throat infection

angine ***f*** **de poitrine** angina pectoris (impairment of the blood vessels in the heart)

angine ***f*** **de Vincent** Vincent's angina (pectoris)

angineux ***m*** **–euse** ***f*** someone with angina pectoris

angiocardographie ***f*** angiocardiography (X-ray examination of the heart)

angiocholécystite ***f*** gall-bladder inflammation

angiocholite ***f*** inflammation of bile ducts from the liver

angiographie ***f*** angiography (X-ray of veins and arteries)

angiologie ***f*** study of blood circulation, associated diseases and treatment

angiome ***m*** angioma (usually benign tumour formed by blood vessels, often a birthmark)

angiopathie ***f*** general term for blood vessel diseases

angioplastie ***f*** surgical repair of impaired artery or vein

angoisse ***f*** anxiety

angor ***m*** angina pectoris

anite ***f*** irritation/infection of the anus

ankylose ***f*** ankylosis (difficulty/ inability to move a joint)

ankylostome ***m*** hookworm

ankylostomiase ***f*****; ankylostomose** ***f*** hookworm disease

anneau ***m*** **de dentition** teething ring

annexectomie ***f*** removal of ovaries or Fallopian tubes

anomalie ***f*** abnormality

anorexie ***f*** **(mentale)** anorexia (nervosa)

anorexie-boulimie ***f*** anorexia-bulimia (overeating disorder)

annulaire ***m*** third finger

anosmie ***f*** loss of sense of smell

antagonistes ***mpl*** antidotes; opposing muscles; opposite organs; opposing systems or organs

antalgique ***m*** analgesic

antécédent ***m*** **(médical)** previous personal or family (medical) history

anthrax ***m*** carbuncle(s)

antiacide ***m*** antacid

antiacnéique ***m*** acne cream

antiallergique ***adj*** allergy alleviating

antiagrégant ***m*** **plaquettaire** anti (blood) platelet aggregation

antiarthritique ***m*** arthritis drug

antiarythmique ***m*** medicine to re-establish regular heartbeat

antiasthmatique ***m*** asthma drug

antibactérien ***m*** **-enne** ***f adj*** antibacterial

antibiothérapie ***f*** treatment through antibiotics

antibiotique ***m and adj*** antibiotic

être/mettre ***v*** **sous antibiotiques** to be/put on antibiotics

anticoagulant ***m*** anticoagulant substance

anticoagulant(e) ***adj*** anticoagulant

anticorps ***m*** antibody

anticorps ***m*** **antiHBS** substance produced by the body of hepatitis B patients

anticonvulsivant(e) ***adj*** anticonvulsant

antidépresseur ***m*** antidepressant

antidiabétique ***m and adj*** medicine which controls diabetes

antidiurétique ***m and adj*** antidiuretic

antidote ***m*** antidote

antidouleur ***m and adj*** painkiller (product); pain relieving

antiémétique ***m and adj*** antiemetic (used to combat side-effects of chemotherapy e.g. vomiting)

antifongique ***m and adj*** antifungal

antigène ***m*** antigen

antigène ***m*** **HBs** substance making up outside part of hepatitis B

antihelminthique ***m and adj*** anthelmintic (drug or agent which destroys parasites)

antihistaminique ***m*** antihistamine (product reducing/preventing allergies)

anti-inflammatoire ***adj*** anti-inflammatory

antimitotique ***f*** antimitotic (chemical substance used in chemotherapy treatment)

antimoustique ***adj*** mosquito repellent (product)

antimycosique ***m*** medicine for treatment of microscopic fungal diseases

antinéoplasique ***m and adj*** anti-neoplasic (anticancer medicine)

antioxydant ***m*** antioxidant

antiprurigineux ***m*** product which eliminates/reduces itching

antipyrétique ***m*** antipyretic drug or agent; febrifuge (medicine which brings down fever)

antipyrétique ***adj*** antipyretic; febrifuge (preventing/reducing fever)

antiscorbutique ***adj*** antiscorbutic (preventing/ curing scurvy)

antisepsie ***f*** antisepsis (the use of antiseptics)

antiséborrhéique ***adj*** agent/product which counters

seborrhoea (excessive sebum discharge)

antiseptique ***m and adj*** antiseptic

antispasmodique ***m and adj*** antispasmodic (medicine: also produced by the body)

antistase ***f*** antistasis (aids circulation)

antitoxine ***f*** antitoxin

antitussif ***m*** cough mixture; cough syrup

antiviral(e) ***adj*** antiviral

antral(e) ***adj*** relating to lower part of stomach

antre du pylore (inflammation ***f*** **de l')** pylorus inflammation

anurèse ***f*****; anurie** ***f*** anuresis; anuria

anurie ***f*** **vraie** kidneys are no longer producing urine

fausse anurie ***f*** kidneys block the urine

anus ***m*** anus

anus ***m*** **artificiel** artificial anus (temporary or permanent)

anxiolytique ***m*** tranquilliser

anxiolytique ***adj*** tranquillising

aorte ***f*** aorta (main artery)

aortographie ***f*** X-ray of the aorta

apaisant(e) ***adj*** soothing (cream, etc.)

apex ***m*** apex (med) (pointed tip/extremity of lung/heart, etc.)

aphasie ***f*** aphasia (total/partial loss of speech or understanding of speech due to brain disease/injury)

aphonie ***f*** total voice loss, generally temporary

aphte ***m*** mouth ulcer

aplasie ***f*** body organ collapse

apnées ***fpl*** **du sommeil** apnoea (involuntary holding of breath, especially during sleep)

aponévrite ***f*** fibrositis

aponévrosite ***f*** **plantaire** inflammation of the sole of the foot

apophyse ***f*** protruding part of a bone

apophysite ***f*** **tibiale antérieure** leg-bone growing pain

appareil ***m*** (medical) appliance; anatomical system

appareil ***m*** **acoustique/auditif** hearing aid

appareil *m* digestif digestive system

appareil *m* orthodontique teeth brace

appareil *m* orthopédique; attelle *f* brace

appareil *m* phonatoire vocal organs

appareil *m* plâtré wet plaster bandage providing support

appareil *m* respiratoire respiratory system

appareil *m* urogénital urogenital system

appareiller *v* to prepare someone, medically, for transport; to fit a person with orthopaedic equipment

appendice *m* anatomical appendage

appendice *m* nasal proboscis

appendicite *f* appendicitis

appendicite *f* aiguë acute appendicitis

appendicite *f* chronique grumbling appendicitis

appendicectomie *f* appendicectomy/appendectomy (surgical removal of appendix)

appétit *m* appetite

apraxie *f* loss of visual memory; inability to move correctly (but not physically handicapped)

après-shampoing *m* hair conditioner

apyrétique *adj* of patient who is no longer feverous

apyrexie *f* absence of fever

aquagym *f* aquagym

arachnoïde *f* arachnoid (middle membrane around the brain and spinal cord)

arc *m* lipoïdique whitish-grey circular liquid patch forming on the eye

armoire *f* à pharmacie medical cabinet

arnica *f* arnica plant

aromathérapie *f* aromatherapy (massage using oils and plant extracts)

arracher *v* to extract

arrêt *m* cardiaque cardiac arrest

arriération *f* mentale mental retardation

artère *f* artery

artériosclérose *f* progressive thickening and hardening of the main arteries

artériographie *f* X-ray of arteries
artériopathie *f* arterial illnesses
artériopathie *f* **diabétique** arterial inflammation due to diabetic condition
artérite *f* inflammation of artery
arthralgie *f* painful joints
arthrite *f* arthritis
arthroplastie *f* surgical repair of impaired joint
arthroplastie *f* **complète de la hanche** hip joint replacement operation
arthroscanner *m* articulation scan
arthroscopie *f* keyhole surgery to examine an artery
arthrose *f* osteoarthritis (degenerative disease of the joints)
articulation *f* joint
articulation *f* **de la hanche** (*or* **articulation coxo-fémorale** *adj*) hip joint
arythmie *f* arrhythmia (irregular heartbeats)
asbestose *f* asbestosis (disease caused by long-term inhalation of asbestos particles)
ascaridiase/-iose *f* roundworm disease
ascaride *f* roundworm
ascite *f* ascites (abnormal build-up of liquid in the stomach)
ascorbique *adj* **(acide)** ascorbic (acid vitamin in citrus fruits)
asexué(e) *adj* sexless/asexual (person)
ASP (see **abdomen sans préparation**)
aspergillose *f* mushroom disease (following consumption of certain fungi)
asphyxie *f* asphyxia
aspirine *f* **(soluble)** (soluble) aspirin
asthénie *f* asthenia (weakness)
asthénie *f* **psychique** impairment of concentration, intelligence and memory
asthénospermie *f* spermatic weakness (linked to male sterility)
asthmatique *adj* asthmatic
asthme *m* asthma
astigmatisme *m* astimagtism (eye defect)
astragale *m* talus (ankle bone supporting the tibia)

astringent ***m and adj*** astringent (of product which checks bleeding)

astrocytome ***m*** brain tumour

ataxie ***f*** ataxy; ataxia (loss of body movement control)

ATB, ATBT abbreviation for antibiotic

atélectasie ***f*** disorder of an area of the lung

athérome ***m*** cholesterol buildup inside artery wall

athérosclose ***f*** artery hardening and thickening due to excessive **athérome**

atlas ***m*** uppermost neck bone

atopie ***f*** form of allergy to pollen, animal hairs, etc.

atrophie ***f*** atrophy (diminution in weight or size of an organ)

attaque ***f*** fit

attaque ***f*** **d'apoplexie** apoplectic fit

atteint(e) ***adj*** affected (by); suffering (from)

attelle ***f*** splint

aubépine ***f*** hawthorn

audiogramme ***m*** audiogram (hearing test)

audiomètre ***m*** audiometer

audiophone ***m*** hearing aid

audition ***f*** hearing

auriculaire ***m*** little finger

auriculaire ***adj*** relating to ear; relating to heart's auricle
extrasystole ***f*** **auriculaire** extrasystole (irregular heartbeat)

auriculothérapie ***f*** aural acupuncture

ausculter ***v*** to listen to heartbeat/breathing, by ear or with a stethoscope

autisme ***m*** autism

autiste ***adj*** of autistic person

autoclave ***m*** autoclave (steam sterilisation apparatus)

autogène ***adj*** autogenous; self-produced

autogreffe ***f*** graft using healthy tissue from patient's own body (see **greffe**)

auto-immunité ***f*** **pathologique** the body's abnormal function of producing substances which attack its own parts and organs

auto-immunité ***f*** **physiologique** the body's

natural function of producing antibodies

autoimmunisation *f* pathologique pathological autoimmunisation

autoimmunisation *f* physiologique physiological autoimmunisation

auto-intoxication *f* auto-intoxication

autolyse *f* autolysis (milder way of saying 'suicide')

automatisme *m* automatism

autonome *adj* independent; autonomous

autopsie *f* autopsy

autoplastie *f* autoplasty (surgical operation using healthy tissue from the patient's body)

autotoxine *f* autotoxin (poisonous substance originating from patient's organism)

autotransfusion *f* auto-blood transfusion (patient's own blood reserve is re-injected during an operation)

autophonie *f* uncomfortable impression in the head of hearing one's own voice

auxiliaire *m*/ *f* médical(e) paramedic

avaler *v* to swallow

avéré(e) *adj* established (illness, by medical tests)

aveugle *m/f* blind man/woman

avant-bras *m* forearm

AVC (see **accident vasculaire cérébral**)

avitaminose *f* illness due to vitamin deficiency

avortement *m* abortion

avortement *m* spontané miscarriage

avortement *m* thérapeutique termination of pregnancy for medical reasons

avulsion *f* dentaire tooth extraction

axis *m* axis (second neck bone)

bacille *m* bacillus (bacterial microbe)

bacille *m* de Koch TB microbe

bactéricide *m and adj* bactericide

bactérie *f* bacterium

bactériologie ***f*** bacteriology
bactériologiste ***m/f*** bacteriologist
bain ***m*** **d'algues/de boue** seaweed/mud bath
bain ***m*** **de bouche/oculaire** mouthwash (rinse)/ eyewash
bain ***m*** **de vapeur** steam bath
bain ***m*** **de soleil** sunbathing
balanite ***f*** inflammation of the tip of the penis
ballonnement ***m*** bloating; distending
bandage ***m*** bandage
bandage ***m*** **herniaire** surgical appliance; truss
bande ***f*** bandage
bande ***f*** **de tissu élastique** elastic support bandage
bande ***f*** **plâtrée** plaster bandage
bande ***f*** **Velpeau®** crêpe bandage
bande ***f*** **élastique** elastic band
bandelette ***f*** dip-test (for substance in blood or urine)
bandelette ***f*** small bandage
bander ***v*** to bandage
banque ***f*** **de peau** skin bank
banque ***f*** **de plasma** plasma bank
banque ***f*** **de sang** blood bank
banque ***f*** **de sperme** sperm bank
barbitémie ***f*** amount of barbituate in the blood
barbiturique ***m*** barbiturate
bardane ***f*** burdock (used for cough syrup)
barème ***m*** **de Glasgow** Glascow Coma scale
barotraumatisme ***m*** ear drum injury due to high altitude, explosions, scuba diving
bascule ***f*** **assise** inclining/ reclining feature on para-medical armchair
basilic ***m*** basil
bassin ***m*** pelvis
petit bassin ***m*** lower pelvis
bassin ***m*** **hygiénique/ de lit** bedpan
bâtonnet ***m*** short pharmaceutical packaging tube; rod (rod shaped structures in the eye)
baume ***m*** balm
baume ***m*** **chauffant** warming balm
bavoir ***m*** bib
bec-de-lièvre ***m*** harelip

belladone *f* belladonna (deadly nightshade)
bégaiement *m* stammering
bénin, -igne *adj* benign
benzodiazépine *f* **(BZD)** benzodiazepine (group of sedatives, including Valium®)
béquille *f* **commune** underarm crutch
béquille *f* **d'avant-bras** forearm crutch
berge *f* edge of a cut/surgical incision/wound
béribéri *m* beriberi
bétabloquant *m*/**bétabloqueur** *m* beta blocker/beta blocking
biceps *m* biceps
bien-être *m* well-being
'bien dans sa tête *f*, **bien dans son corps** *m*' 'healthy mind, healthy body'
bicarbonate de sodium *m* sodium bicarbonate
bifurcation *f* **aortique** aortic split (near stomach)
bile *f* bile
bilieux –ieuse *adj* bilious
bilharziose *f* bilharzia ('worms')
bilirubine *f* bilirubin (one of bile's constituent substances)
bilirubinémie *f* the amount of bile in the blood
biochimie *f* biochemistry
biodégradabilité *f* biodegradability
biologie *f* biology
biométrie *f* body measurements and weight
biopsie *f* biopsy
fragment *m* **biopsique** sample for biopsy
biorythme *m* biorhythm
biscuit *m* **pour bébé** rusk
bistouri *m* bistoury (surgical scalpel)
bithérapie *f* treatment using two medicines
blennoragie *f* gonorrhea
blépharite *f* blepharitis (eyelid inflammation)
blesser *v* to injure/hurt/wound
se blesser *v* to injure/hurt/wound oneself
blessure *f* wound/injury
blessure *f* **béante** gaping wound
bleu *m* bruise
bleu *m* **de méthylène** methylene blue (antiseptic)
bloc *m* **cardiaque** cardiac block (pulse blockage)

bloc *m* opératoire operating theatre

blocage *m* blockage

blocage *m* intestinal intestinal blockage

blocage *m* de mémoire memory block

bobo *m* small cut/sore (used when speaking to young children)

boîte *f* crânienne skull

boîter *v* to limp

bol *m* bolus; large pill

bombe *f* aérosol aerosol can/ spray

bombe *f* au cobalt cobalt therapy unit; telecobalt machine

bombement *m* swelling (esp. forehead)

bosse *f* lump; bump

botulisme *m* botulism (serious food poisoning through poor food conservation)

bouche-à-bouche *m* mouth-to-mouth (resuscitation)

bouillie *f* de sulphate de barium barium sulphate and water meal (for stomach opacity prior to stomach X-rays)

bouillir *v* to boil

bouleau *m* silver birch

boulimie *f* bulimia

boulimique *adj* bulimic

bourdonnement *m* d'oreilles ringing or buzzing in ears

bourgeon *m* pimple; spot (formed on a healing cut/ wound)

bourrache *f* officinale borage (plant)

bourrage *m* alimentaire food wedged between teeth

bourrelet *m* de chair roll of flesh (pads under the fingers)

bourrelet *m* de graisse roll of fat

bout *m* tip (finger, nose etc.)

bouton *m* pimple; spot

bouton *m* d'acné acne spot

bouton *m* de fièvre cold sore

boutonneux –euse *adj* pimply; spotty

BPCO (see **broncho-pneumopathie chronique obstructive**)

BPM (battement de cœur par minute) heartbeat rate per minute; pulse

brachialgie ***f*** pain in the arm
bradycardie ***f*** bradycardia (abnormally slow pulse)
bradypnée ***f*** abnormally slow breathing rate
brancard ***m*** stretcher
brancardier ***m*** stretcher-bearer
bras ***m*** arm
bras ***m*** **cassé** broken arm
brochage ***m*** pinning (of fractured bone)
broche ***f*** pin (support)
bronche ***f*** bronchial tube
bronchectasie ***f*** widening of the bronchial tubes
bronchioles ***fpl*** bronchioles (small tubes branching off the bronchial tubes)
bronchiolite ***f*** bronchialitis (potentially serious infection of bronchioles, with wheezing symptoms, in babies)
bronchite ***f*** bronchitis
bronchodilatateur ***m*** bronchodilator (treats asthma)
broncho-pneumopathie ***f*** **chronique obstructive** chronic bronchopneumonia
bronchospasme ***m*** contraction of the bronchial tubes
bronzage ***m*** suntanning
brucellose ***f*** brucellosis; undulant fever; Malta fever
brûler ***v*** **to** burn
brûlure ***f*** burn
brûlure ***f*** **d'eau bouillante** scald with boiling water
brûlure ***f*** **du premier/ deuxième/troisième degré** first/second/third degree burn
brûlure ***f*** **de cigarette** cigarette burn
brûlures ***fpl*** **d'estomac** heartburn
buccal(e) ***adj*** buccal; concerning the mouth
  cavité ***f*** **buccale** inside of the mouth
  respiration ***f*** **buccale** breathing through the mouth
bulbe ***m*** bulbous-shaped organ or organ part
bulbe ***m*** **pileux** hair bulb
bulbe ***m*** **de l'oeil** main part of the eye
bulbe ***m*** **rachidien** medulla oblongata (spinal bulb at bottom of brain)
bulle ***f*** **dermatologique** skin blister

bulle *f* pulmonaire permanently air-filled lung cavity

bulleux –euse ***adj*** blistering

bursite *f* bursitis (inflammation of a bursa/fluid filled sac)

BZD (abbreviation of benzodiazépine)

cachet *m* à croquer chewable tablet

cachet *m* soluble soluble tablet

cadre *m* colique the four parts of the large intestine which form a square

caecum *m* caecum (first part of the large intestine)

cage *f* thoracique thoracic/rib cage

caillot *m* (blood) clot

cal *m* callus

calamine *f* calamine

lotion *f* calmante à la calamine calamine lotion

calcanéen -éenne ***adj*** relating to the calcaneum(heel bone)

épine *f* calcanéenne pointed bone abnormality below the calcaneum

calcanéum *m* calcaneum (heel bone)

calcémie *f* amount of calcium in the blood

calcifiant(e) ***adj*** producing calcium deposits

pancréatite *f* calcifiante illness which calcifies the pancreas

calcification *f* calcification

calcium *m* calcium

calcul *m* calculus; stone formed in body

calcul *m* biliaire gall stone; bile stone

calcul *m* rénal kidney stone

calleux -euse ***adj*** callous

callosité *f* callus

calmant *m* antidouleur painkiller

calmant *m* tranquillisant sedative tranquilliser

calmant *m* pour coliques infantiles gripe water

calotte *f* crânienne dome of the skull

calvitie *f* baldness

camomille *f* allemande German camomile

canal *m* canal; duct

canal *m* anal rectum

canal *m* biliaire bile duct
canal *m* carpien carpal canal (duct containing tendons linked to finger bones)
canal *m* déférent vas deferens (spermatic duct from testicle to uretha)
canal *m* lacrymal tear duct
canal *m* thoracique thoracic duct
cancer *m* cancer
cancer *m* de la peau skin cancer
cancer *m* de l'estomac stomach cancer
cancer *m* de l'œsphage throat cancer
cancer *m* du col de l'utérus cervical (womb) cancer
cancer *m* du poumon lung cancer
cancer *m* du rein kidney cancer
cancer *m* du sang leukaemia
cancer *m* du sein breast cancer
cancéreux –euse *adj* cancerous; person suffering from cancer
cancérigène *adj* cancer-producing
cancérologue *m/f* cancer specialist
cancérophobie *f* obsessional fear of having cancer
Candida albicans *m* Candida albicans (fungus that causes thrush)
candidose *f* candidosis; moniliasis; thrush (white patchy infection of the mouth and throat and/or the vagina)
canine *f* canine tooth
canne *f* walking stick
canne *f* anglaise forearm crutch
canne *f* blanche white stick
capillaire *m* capillary
lotion *f* capillaire hair lotion
capital santé (see **accroître son capital santé)**
capital *m* soleil body's capacity to resist long-term harmful effects of sunbathing
capital *m* soleil épuisé exhausted (used up) capacity to resist harmful effects of sunbathing
capital *m* soleil réduit reduced (time) capacity to resist harmful effects of sunbathing

capsule *f* capsule; pouch separating different body organs

carcinome *m* carcinoma (cancers of skin, digestive tract and lung)

cardiaque *adj* cardiac

cardio-vasculaire *adj* cardiovascular

cardiogramme *m* cardiogram (record of heart muscle activity)

cardiographe *m* cardiograph (instrument which measures heart muscle activity)

cardiologie *f* cardiology (study/ treatment of heart and blood circulation)

cardiologue *m/f* cardiologist (heart and blood circulation specialist)

cardiopathie *f* heart disease

cardiomyopathie *f* cardiomyopathy (heart muscle disease)

coronaropathie *f* heart artery disease

cardiochirurgien(ne) *m/f* heart surgeon

cardite *f* carditis (inflammation of heart membranes)

carence *f* **en vitamines** vitamin deficiency

carie *f* tooth or bone decay

carotène *m* carotene (Vitamin A orange or red pigment)

carotide *f* carotid (either of two arteries taking blood from the heart to neck and head)

carpe *m* carpus; wrist bones

carrefour *m* **laryngé** cross-over junction between the windpipe and alimentary canal

cartilage *m* cartilage

caryotype *m* karyotype (number and chromosome types in a cell nucleus)

cas *m* case

casser *v* to break

cassé(e) *adj* broken

cassis *m* blackcurrant

castration *f* castration

catalepsie *f* catalepsy; trance

cataplasme *m* poultice; cataplasm

cataplasme *m* **de moutarde** mustard poultice

cataplasme *m* **sinapisé** mustard poultice

cataracte ***f*** cataract
catarrhe ***m*** catarrh
catgut ***m*** catgut
cathartique ***m and adj*** cathartic
cathéter ***m*** catheter
cathétérisme ***m*** catheterisation (using catheter to inject into veins)
cauchemar ***m*** nightmare
cautère ***m*** cauterisation (with electrically heated instrument)
cautérisation ***f*** cauterisation
cautériser ***v*** to cauterise
cavité ***f*** cavity
cavité ***f*** **abdominale** abdominal cavity
cavité ***f*** **articulaire** bone socket
cavité ***f*** **nasale** nasal cavity
cavité ***f*** **pleurale** rib cavity
cavité ***f*** **pulpaire** (tooth) pulp cavity
cavum ***m*** rear of nose joining top of throat
CEC (circulation extra-corporelle) ***f*** external electric pumps and tubes which maintain blood circulation during open-heart surgery
cécité ***f*** blindness
ceinture ***f*** **herniaire** truss
ceinture ***f*** **orthopédique** surgical corset
ceinture ***f*** **pelvienne** pelvic (bone) girdle
cellule ***f*** cell
cellule ***f*** **sanguine** blood cell
cellulite ***f*** cellulite; cellulitis (inflammation of cell tissue)
céphaléé ***f*** cephalalgia; headache
céphalique ***adj*** relating to the head
céphalo-rachidien(ne) ***adj*** cerebrospinal
liquide ***m*** **céphalo-rachidien** cerebrospinal fluid
céphalosporine ***f*** antibiotic group (closely related to penicillin)
cerclage ***m*** **d'un os cassé** hooping repair to broken bone (with metal wire)
cerclage ***m*** **du col de l'utérus** cervical cerclage (surgical procedure performed during pregnancy where cervix is sewn closed)
cerebral(e) ***adj*** cerebral
cernes ***mpl*** rings (under the eyes)
cérumen ***m*** earwax

cerveau ***m*** brain
cervelet ***m*** cerebellum (the back of the brain)
cervicalgie ***f*** neck pain
césarienne ***f*** caesarean
chalazion ***m*** chalazion (small abscess in/on eyelid)
chambre ***f*** **à coucher** bedroom
chambre ***f*** **de travail préparatoire à l'accouchement** labour room
champ ***m*** **opératoire** uncovered body area, ready for surgery
champ ***m*** **visuel** field of vision
champignon ***m*** fungus; mushroom
champignon ***m*** **comestible** edible mushroom
champignon ***m*** **hallucinogène** hallucinogenic mushroom; magic mushroom
champignon ***m*** **vénéneux** toadstool; poisonous mushroom
chancre ***m*** **mou; chancrelle** ***f*** chancroid; soft chancre (VD groin ulcer)
chancre ***m*** **syphilitique** chancre
charbon ***m*** **activé** activated charcoal/carbon (for adsorptive properties)
chauffe-biberon ***m*** baby bottle warmer
charge ***f*** **virale** virus count in the blood
chauve ***adj*** bald
chéloïde ***f*** fibrous swelling on a scar
cheveux ***mpl*** hair
chute ***f*** **des cheveux** hair loss
cheville ***f*** ankle
cheville ***f*** **foulée** twisted ankle
chiendent ***m*** couch grass
chimiothérapie ***f*** chemotherapy
chiropracteur ***m*** chiropractor (usually not a doctor)
chiropractie ***f*** chiropractic (manipulation of the joints)
chirurgie ***f*** surgery
chirurgie ***f*** **cardiaque** heart surgery
chirurgie ***f*** **conservatrice du sein** cancer surgery which conserves the affected breast
chirurgie ***f*** **dentaire** dental surgery work

chirurgie ***f*** **esthétique** cosmetic surgery

chirurgie ***f*** **maxillaire** jaw surgery

chirurgie ***f*** **ophtalmique** eye surgery

chirurgie ***f*** **réparatrice** reconstruction surgery

chirurgien(ne) ***m/f*** surgeon

CHIVA ***f*** **(cure conservatrice et hyémodynamique de l'insuffisance veineuse en ambulatoire)** varicose-vein operation as outpatient

chlamydia ***f*** chlamidia (small parasitic bacterium)

choc (médical) ***m*** medical shock (reaction, possibly fatal)

choc ***m*** **anesthésique** shock due to anaestheics

choc ***m*** **anaphylactique** anaphylactic shock

choc ***m*** **cardiogènique** cardiac shock

choc ***m*** **électrique** electric shock

choc ***m*** **hypovolémique** shock due to sudden drop in blood pressure

choc ***m*** **nerveux** nervous shock

choc ***m*** **opératoire** post-operative shock

choc ***m*** **psychologique** psychological shock

choc ***m*** **septique** toxic shock

cholécystectomie ***f*** cholycystectomy (surgical removal of the gall bladder)

cholécystographie ***f*** X-ray of the gall bladder

cholécystite ***f*** gall bladder inflammation

choléra ***m*** cholera

cholestase ***f*** bile blockage

cholestéatome ***m*** ear tumour (following repeated ear infections)

cholestérol ***m*** cholesterol

cholestérolémie ***f*** cholesterol amount in the blood

chondropathie ***f*** cartilage disorders

choquer ***v*** to shake, to shock

chorée ***f*** **de Huntington** Huntington's chorea (with progressive dementia)

chorée ***f*** **de Sydenham** Sydenham's chorea

chorion ***m*** chorion (outermost membrane around an embryo)

choroïde *f* eyeball membrane
choroïdite *f* choroiditis (inflammation of the eye membrane)
chromosome *m* chromosome
chronique *adj* chronic
chute *f* **des reins** small of the back
chyle *m* chyle (whitish digestive fluid in small intestine)
cicatrice *f* scar
cicatrisant *m* healing product
cicatrisant(e) *adj* healing
cicatriser *v* to heal; form a scar
cil *m* eyelash
circulation *f* **sanguine** blood circulation
cinétique *f* **du coeur** study of the heart's kinetics
circonscrire *v* **une infection** to contain an infection
circoncision *f* circumcision
circulation *f* **collatérale** blood circulation bypassing main artery or vein
cirrhose *f* **du foie** cirrhosis of the liver
ciseaux *mpl* **à ongles** nail scissors
civière *f* stretcher
clairance *f* kidney's ability to filter waste from the blood
claudication *f* limp
claustrophobie *f* claustrophobia
cliché *m* X-ray
clitoris *m* clitoris
cloison *f* **du nez** nasal septum (between the nostrils)
clavicule *f* clavicle
clone *m* clone
cloque *f* blister
cloquer *v* to blister
clou *m* boil
coagulant *m* coagulant
coagulation *f* coagulation
cochlée *f* cochlea (snail-shaped cavity inside the ear)
implant *m* **cochléaire** minute hearing aid implanted in the ear
coccyx *m* coccyx
codage *m* **génétique** genetic code
coeur *m* heart
col *m* neck
col du fémur *m* **cassé** broken neck of the femur
col *m* **de l'utérus** cervix
col *m* **de la vessie** neck of the bladder

colibacillose ***f*** colibacillosis (bacterial infection in large intestine)

colique ***f*** colic

colique ***f*** **biliaire** biliary colic

colique ***f*** **hépatique** hepatic (liver) colic

colique ***f*** **néphrétique** renal (kidney) colic

colique ***f*** **salivaire** colic in the jaw and cheek

coliques ***fpl*** gripes (violent stomach pains)

colique ***f*** **de plomb** lead poisoning colic

colique ***adj*** relating to the colon

colite ***f*** colitis (inflammation of the colon)

collation ***f*** light meal

collet ***m*** neck area inside mouth (around teeth and gums)

côlon ***m*** colon (major part of large intestine)

côlon ***m*** **sigmoïde**; **côlon** ***m*** **pelvien** sigmoid colon (curved intestine just before the rectum)

coloniser ***v*** to colonise (to be overrun by/infested by)

colopathie ***f*** **fonctionnelle** irritable bowel syndrome

coloscopie ***f*** coloscopy (examination by optic fibres inside the colon)

colonne ***f*** **vertébrale** spinal column

colostomie ***f*** colostomy (surgical operation to replace part of the colon, bypassing the anus)

collagène ***m and adj*** collagen (major structural protein)

colposcopie ***f*** colposcopyvaginal and neck of the womb examination)

colostrum ***m*** colostrum (first post-natal breast secretion)

coma ***m*** coma

coma ***m*** **diabétique** diabetic coma

coma ***m*** **léger** comatose with poor response

coma ***m*** **vigile** comatose with good response

coma ***m*** **profond** deep coma

coma ***m*** **dépassé** brain-dead

comitialité ***f*** severe epilepsy

comédon ***m*** blackhead

comédogène ***adj*** comedogenic (blocks the pores)
comestible ***adj*** edible
commotion ***f*** **cérébrale** concussion
commotion ***f*** **électrique** electric shock
commotion ***f*** **mentale** mental shock
commotionné ***adj*** in a state of shock; concussed
communiquer ***v*** **une maladie** to spread/pass on an illness
compatibilité ***f*** compatibility
compensation ***f*** compensation (helpful or curative physiological modification or psychological reaction)
compère-loriot ***m*** sty(e)
complément ***m*** **alimentaire** complementary foodstuff
compliance ***f*** elasticity; suppleness
complications ***fpl*** complications
complication ***f*** **mineure** minor complication
compresse ***f*** compress
compresse ***f*** **antiseptique** antiseptic compress
compresse ***f*** **de gaze** gauze compress
compresse ***f*** **'physiopack'** hot or cold compress
compressif –ive ***adj*** compressive
comprimé (cp) ***m*** tablet
comprimé ***m*** **pelliculé** coated tablet
comprimé ***m*** **sublingual** tablet taken under the tongue
compte-gouttes ***m*** dropper/ pipette
conception ***f*** conception
concrétion ***f*** concretion (stony mass formed in body)
concrétion ***f*** **calcaire** calcareous stones (in the body)
condamné(e) ***adj*** terminally ill
condamner ***v*** to abandon hope
condensation ***f*** **d'un os** increase in bone density
conditions ***fpl*** **de conservation** conservation stipulations
conditionneur ***m*** hair conditioner
conduction ***f*** conduction (of blood)
conduit ***m*** duct

condylome ***m*** small tumour (benign) near genitals
condylome ***m*** **acuminé** sexually transmitted tumour (benign) near genitals
confusion ***f*** **mentale** mental confusion/disorder (temporary)
congenital(e) ***adj*** congenital
congestif –ive ***adj*** (organ) containing too much blood
congestion ***f*** congestion
congestion ***f*** **cérébrale** stroke
congestion ***f*** **pulmonaire** lung congestion
conisation ***f*** surgical removal of part of cervix of the womb
conjonctive ***f*** eyelid membrane
conjonctivite ***f*** conjunctivitis
connaissance ***f*** consciousness
consanguinité ***f*** consanguinity
conscience ***f*** awareness; consciousness
perdre/reprendre ***v*** **connaissance/conscience** to lose/regain consciousness
conseiller ***v*** to advise; to recommend
consentement ***m*** consent
consolidation ***f*** setting (of fracture)
consolider ***v*** to set (a fractured bone)
constatation ***f*** **(clinique)** (clinical) observation
constipation ***f*** constipation
constipé(e) ***adj*** constipated
constitution ***f*** constitution
contactologie ***f*** study of (spectacle) lenses and contact lenses
contagion ***f*** contagion; contagiousness
contamination ***f*** contamination
contaminer ***v*** to contaminate
contaminé(e) ***adj*** contaminated
contention ***f*** strong support (includes plasters, support stockings and splints)
continence ***f*** bowels and bladder performing correctly; sexual abstinence
contraception ***f*** contraception
contraceptif ***m*** contraceptive
contraction ***f*** **musculaire** cramp
contractions ***fpl*** **utérines** childbirth contractions
contracture ***f*** spasm
contre-indication ***f*** contraindication

contrepoison ***m*** antidote

contrôle ***m*** **des naissances** birth control

contrôle ***m*** **d'alcoolémie** testing alcohol percentage in the blood

contusion ***f*** bruise

contusionner ***v*** to bruise

contusionné(e) ***adj*** bruised

convalescence ***f*** convalescence

convulsions ***fpl*** **fébriles** feverish convulsions

coqueluche ***f*** whooping cough

cor ***m*** corn

corde ***f*** **spinale** spinal cord

corde ***f*** **vocale** vocal cord

cordon ***m*** **médullaire** spinal cord

cordon ***m*** **ombilical** umbilical cord

cordon ***m*** **spermatique** spermatic cord spermatic cord (nerves, ducts, blood vessels going to the testicles)

cornée ***f*** cornea

cornet ***m*** skull bone behind the nose

coronaire ***adj*** coronary

coronarien(ne) ***adj*** patient with coronary artery disorder

coronarographie ***f*** X-ray of coronary arteries

corps ***m*** body; part of the anatomy

corps ***m*** **étranger** foreign body

corps ***m*** **jaune** yellow body (hormone-secreting structure developed in ovary)

corps ***m*** **vitré** vitreous body (eye)

corpulence ***f*** corpulence; stoutness

de faible/forte/moyenne corpulence ***f*** of slight/stout/ medium build

corriger ***v*** to correct (vision, etc.)

corrompre ***v*** to contaminate (blood, etc.)

cortex ***m*** cortex (external part of an organ)

cortex ***m*** **cérébral** cerebral cortex

corticoïde ***m*** corticoid (substance produced by gland above the kidney); medicinal group treating inflammations and allergies

corticothérapie ***f*** course of corticoid treatment

cortisone *f* cortisone
coryza *m* coryza; head cold
coryza *m* **spasmodique des foins** hay fever
cotyle *m* bone socket receiving another bone (esp. hip socket receiving top of thigh bone)
côte *f* rib
côte *f* **cassée** broken rib
cou *m* neck
cou-de-pied *m* instep
couche-culotte *f* disposable nappy
couche *f* **jetable** disposable nappy
couche *f* **pour incontinents** incontinence pad
couches, *fpl* **en** in confinement; childbirth
couches *fpl* **pénibles** difficult labour
coude *m* elbow
couenne *f* (inflammatory) membrane
coup *m* **de chaleur** heatstroke
coup *m* **de froid** cold; chill
attraper *v* **un coup de froid** to catch a cold/chill
coup *m* **de pompe** exhaustion
avoir *v* **un coup de pompe** to feel drained/exhausted
coup *m* **de soleil** sunburn
coupe *f* sectioned (of usually infected body part) area for microscope examination
coupe-faim *m* appetite suppressant
couperose *f* red acne; rosacea (swollen, visible blood vessels)
coupole *f* **diaphragmatique** diaphragm (muscle area separating chest from stomach)
coupe *f* **tranversale** cross-section
coupure *f* cut
courbatures *fpl* aches and pains; stiffness
couronne *f* crown (of tooth)
couronne *f* **dentaire** capping (of tooth)
coussin *m* **chauffant anti-rhumatisme (à champ magnétique)** heated, magnetised cushion for rheumatism
coussin *m* **de positionnement** small of the back cushion support

coussin *m* de voyage travel neck rest cushion

couturier *m* sartorial (thigh) muscle

couveuse *f* incubator

couverture *f* chauffante electric blanket

coxalgie *f* TB of the hip

coxarthrose *f* arthritis of the hip

crampe *f* cramp

crampe *f* d'estomac stomach cramp

crampe *f* au mollet cramp in the calf

crampe *f* de l'écrivain writer's cramp

crâne *m* skull

créatine *f* creatine (protein metabolism produced in muscles)

CPK *f* (créatine phosphokanise) substance in blood which increases with muscle disorder

créatinémie *f* amount of creatine in the blood

crème *f* cream

crème *f* antirougeurs cream for red skin

crème *f* antiseptique antiseptic cream

crème *f* contre les rougeurs nappy rash cream

crème *f* hydratante moisturiser; moisturising cream

crème *f* solaire suntan lotion

crème *f* pour bébés baby cream

crème *f* pour les mains hand cream

crème *f* pour le visage face cream

crépitant *adj* crackling/rattling (of sound), detected by stethoscope indicating or with certain lung diseases

crépitation *f* crepitation; crackling/rattling

crépitation *f* articulaire articulary crepitation

crépitation *f* osseuse bony crepitation

crépitation *f* pulmonaire; (lung) crepitation

crête *f* du tibia edge of the shin bone

crétinisme *m* cretinism

Creutzfeld-Jakob, maladie *f* de Creutzfeld-Jakob disease

crevasser *v* to chap
(se) crevasser *v* to become chapped
crever *v* **un abcès** to burst an abscess
crise *f* attack; crisis; fit
crise d'appendicite *f* attack of appendicitis
crise *f* **d'asthme** asthma attack
crise *f* **cardiaque** heart attack
crise *f* **d'épilepsie** epileptic fit
crise *f* **de foie** bilious attack; severe indigestion
crise *f* **de toux** coughing fit
cristallin *m* crystalline lens (in eye)
Crohn, maladie *f* **de** Crohn's disease (chronic intestinal inflammation)
croquer *v* to crunch
crosse *f* **de l'aorte** semi-circular part of the aorta
CRP *f* **(protéine C réactive)** creative protein (excessive amounts of this substance in blood is an indicator of many illnesses)
croup *m* croup (larynx inflammation with hard cough)
croup *m*, **faux** spasmodic croup
croissance *f* development (of illness); growth/development (child, adolescent, etc.)
croûte *f* scab
crural(e) *adj* of/concerning the thigh
cruralgie *f* thigh pain
cryothérapie *f* cryotherapy (low-temperature treatments)
crypte *f* crypt (small concave area of organ)
cryptorchidie *f* congenital testicle disorder (felt in stomach)
cubitus *m* ulna (forearm bone)
cuillerée *f* **à café /à soupe** teaspoonful/tablespoonful
cuir chevelu *m* scalp
cuisine *f* **allégée/légère** low-fat cooking
cuisine *f* **minceur** low-calorie foods
cuisse *f* thigh
cuivre *m* copper
curare *m* curare (an anaesthetic)
cure *f* course of treatment
cure *f* **d'amaigrissement** slimming course
cure *f* **de sommeil** sleep therapy

cure *f* de thalassothérapie seawater therapy

cure *f* thermale spa course of treatment

cure *f* de désintoxication treatment for alcoholism or drug addiction

cure-dents *m* toothpick

curettage *m* curettage

curette *f* curette; scraper

Cushing, syndrome *m* de Cushing's syndrome (overproduction of gluocorticoids)

Cushing, maladie *f* de Cushing's disease

cyanose *f* cyanosis (bluish skin due to lack of oxygen)

cyclothymie *f* manic depression

cyanosé(e) *adj* of person affected by cyanosis; of body area affected by cyanosis

cystite *f* cystitis (bladder inflammation)

cystoscopie *f* cystoscopy (internal examination of bladder using fiberscope)

cytologie *f* cytology (study of cells)

cytolyse *f* destruction of cells

cytoponction *f* taking of cell samples for analysis

daltonien(ne) *adj* colour-blind

daltonisme *m* colour blindness

danse *f* de St Guy St Vitus dance

date *f* limite de conservation best-before date (foodstuffs)

déambulateur *m* walking frame; zimmer frame

déambulation *f* aimless wandering (of the mentally ill)

débander *v* to unbandage

débilité *f* mentale mental deficiency

déboîter *v* to dislocate

décéder *v* to die

décès *m* death

décharge *f* électrique electric shock

déchirer *v* to tear

(se) déchirer *v* un muscle to tear a muscle

déchirure *f* tear; laceration

décibel *m* decibel
90-120 dB: sons *mpl* nocifs 90–120 dB: harmful noises

décollement *m* abnormal detachment (of organism, etc.)

décollement ***m*** **du placenta** detachment of placenta from the uterus

décollement ***m*** **de la rétine** detachment of the retina

décoller ***v*** to lose weight quickly *(informal)*

(se) décoller ***v*** to become abnormally detached

décongestif ***m*** decongestant

décongestif –ive ***adj*** decongestant

décongestionner ***v*** to relieve congestion

décontractant ***m*** relaxation drug

décroissance ***f*** dimunition

décubitus ***m*** lying down position

décubitus ***m*** **dorsal** lying down on the back position

décubitus ***m*** **latéral** lying down on the side position

décubitus ***m*** **ventral** lying down on the front/stomach position

défaillance ***f*** feeling of sickness or faintness (general meaning); fault in function or failure of an organ

défaillance ***f*** **cardiaque** heart failure

défaillance ***f*** **de mémoire** lapse in memory

défécation ***f*** defecation

défenses ***fpl*** **immunitaires** immune defence system

défibrillateur ***m*** defibrillator (electrical apparatus to revive heart)

défibrillation ***f*** defibrillation

déficience ***f*** **mentale** mental deficiency

déficience ***f*** **immunitaire** immunodeficiency

déficience ***f*** **musculaire** muscular insufficiency

déficient(e) ***adj*** **mental (e)** ***adj*** of mentally handicapped person

déficient(e) ***adj*** **visuel(le)** ***adj*** of visually handicapped person

déficient(e) ***adj*** **moteur** of physically handicapped person

déficit ***m*** **en fer** iron deficiency

déficit ***m*** **intellectuel** mental defect

déficit ***m*** **en magnésium** magnesium deficiency

déficit *m* psychologique psychological defect

défilé *m* narrow passage between two bones or organs

défilé *m* costo-claviculaire narrow passage between first rib and clavicle

déformation *f* deformation

dégagement *m* delivery (at childbirth)

dégager *v* to clear (nose, throat, chest, etc.)

(se) dégarnir *v* to go bald; to get thin on top

dégénération *f* degeneration

dégénéré(e) *adj* degenerate; mentally handicapped person

dégénérescence *f* deterioration

dégénérescence *f* calcaire calcareous sedimentation of tissue/organ, blocking their function

dégénérescence *f* maculaire liée à l'âge (DMLA) macular degeneration (deterioration of the most important part of the retina)

déglobulisation *f* dimunition of red corpuscles

déglutir *v* to swallow

déglutition *f* deglutition; act of swallowing

degré *m* degree

degré Baumé *m* degree Baumé (density scale for liquids)

déjection *f* evacuation; defecation

déjections *fpl* excrement

délire *m* alcoolique alcoholic mania

délire *m* hallucinatoire hallucinatory delirium

délire *m* de persécution persecution mania

delirium *m* tremens delirium tremens (psychosis caused by chronic alcoholism)

deltoïde *m* deltoid (shoulder muscle)

démangeaison *f* itch; itching

démanger *v* to itch

démaquiller *v* to stop treatment before check-up to give real state of health

démence *f* madness/insanity; dementia

dément(e) *adj* of demented person

démettre *v* to dislocate

(se) démettre ***v*** **le poignet/ l'épaule** to dislocate one's wrist/shoulder
démis(e) ***adj*** dislocated; out of joint
dengue ***f*** dengue fever (tropical disease causing acute joint pains)
déminéralisation ***f*** abnormal calcium loss (in bones)
densité ***f*** **mammaire** mammary density (mammography factor)
densité ***f*** **osseuse** calcium level in a bone
densitométrie ***f*** **osseuse** measurement of calcium level in bones
dent ***f*** tooth
dent ***f*** **artificielle** artificial tooth
dent ***f*** **creuse** hollow tooth
dent ***f*** **définitive/de remplacement** second/ permanent tooth
dent ***f*** **gâtée** bad tooth
dent ***f*** **de lait** milk tooth
dent ***f*** **de sagesse** wisdom tooth
dents ***fpl*** **de derrière** back teeth
dents ***fpl*** **du fond** back teeth
dents ***fpl*** **de devant** front teeth
dents ***fpl*** **du bas** lower teeth
dents ***fpl*** **du haut** upper teeth
dentaire ***adj*** dental
  art ***m*** **dentaire** dental technique
  formule ***f*** **dentaire** dentition (type, number and arrangement of teeth)
dentier ***m*** denture; dental plate
dentifrice ***m*** toothpaste
dentifrice ***m*** **fluoré** fluoride toothpaste
  pâte ***f*** **dentifrice** toothpaste
  poudre ***f*** **dentifrice** tooth powder
dentine ***f*** dentine (bony substance forming the tooth)
dentiste ***m/f*** dentist
dentisterie ***f*** dentistery
dentition ***f*** dentition
denture ***f*** set of teeth
dénutrition ***f*** **légère** slight undernourishment (5–10 per cent weight loss)
dénutrition ***f*** **modérée** moderate undernourishment (10–15 per cent weight loss)
dénutrition ***f*** **sévère** severe undernourishment (over 15 per cent weight loss)

déodorant *m* antisudoral antiperspirant

déontologie *f* médicale medical ethics

départment *m* d'oto-rhino-laryngologie ear, nose and throat department

dépasser *v* to exceed

dépendance *f* addiction (to a drug)

dépendant(e) *adj* dependent

dépendante, personne âgée *f* elderly dependent person

dépilatoire *m* depilatory (agent that removes unwanted hair)

dépiler *v* to cause hair loss; to remove hair

dépistage *m* screening test

dépistage *m* du SIDA AIDS screening

dépister *v* to detect; to screen

(se) déplacer *v* to move around

(se) déplacer rapidement *v* to move around quickly

(se) déplacer *v* une articulation to put a joint out

déplâtrage *m* taking a plaster cast off a limb

dépôt *m* deposit

dépressif –ive *adj* depressive

dépression *f* depression

dépression *f* légère/modérée slight/moderate depression

dépression *f* masquée depression without usual symptoms

dépression *f* nerveuse nervous breakdown

dépression *f* névrotique neurotic depression

dépression *f* opératoire post-operative depression

dépression *f* réactionnelle unusually serious depression following unpleasant occurrence/event

dermatite *f* dermatitis (skin inflammation)

dermatologie *f* dermatology

dermatologiste *m/f* dermatologist; skin specialist

dermatose *f* dermatosis (skin disease)

dermatose squameuse *f* scaly skin disease

dermatophytose *f* skin disease/dermatosis following consumption of non-edible fungus

dermite ***f*** inflammation of the skin

dermite ***f*** **séborrhéique du nourrisson** skin redness and fatty scabs on babies

désaxé(e) ***adj*** out-of-true bone

descente ***f*** **d'organe** prolapse of an organ

désensiblisation ***f*** desensitisation (to allergies)

déséquilibre ***m*** imbalance (between parts of anatomy usually same size: lungs, feet, fingers,etc.); unbalance (mental)

déshabiller ***v*** **complètement** to strip off completely (to remove all of one's clothes)

déshabiller ***v*** **jusqu' à la ceinture** to strip off to the waist

déshydratation ***f*** dehydration

déshydraté(e) ***adj*** dehydrated

desinfectant ***m and adj*** disinfectant

désinfecter ***v*** to disinfect

désinfection ***f*** disinfection

désintoxication ***f*** detoxification

désintoxiquer ***v*** to detoxify

désodé(e) ***adj*** sodium free

désordre ***m*** **fonctionnel/hépatique** functional/liver disorder

désorganisation ***f*** **(d'un malade)** patient's lack of concentration and precision

détente ***f*** relaxation

détersion ***f*** thorough cleaning and disinfection (of cut)

détresse ***f*** **respiratoire** severe respiratory difficulties (reanimation required)

déviation ***f*** inversion or abnormal position (of an organ)

déviation ***f*** **de la cloison nasale** displacement of the nasal septum

déviation ***f*** **de l'utérus** displacement of uterus

déviation ***f*** **de la colonne vertébrale** curvature of the spine

dextrose ***m*** dextrose

diabète ***m*** diabetes

diabète ***m*** **insipide** insipid diabetes (deficiency of hormone regulating kidney)

diabète ***m*** **sucré** diabetes mellitus (sweet diabetes),

insulinodépendant(e) ***adj*** diabetes mellitus requiring daily insulin injections; insulin-dependent **person**

diabétique ***adj*** diabetic

diabétique ***m/f*** person suffering from diabetes

diabétologue ***m/f*** diabetes specialist

diagnostic ***m*** diagnostic

recherche ***f*** **diagnostique** diagnostic test/observations

diagnostiquer ***v*** to diagnose

dialyse ***f*** **rénale** renal dialysis

dialyseur ***m*** dialyser

diaphragme ***m*** diaphragm

diarrhée ***f*** diarrhoea

diastole ***f*** **(see also systole)** diastole (intervals between heart contractions when the chambers fill with blood)

DID (abbreviation of diabète insulinodépendant, see definition above)

diète ***f*** diet

diététicien(ne) ***m/f*** dietician

diététique ***adj*** diet (food, drink)

difformité ***f*** abnormality

diffus(e) ***adj*** diffuse; not localised

digérer ***v*** to digest

digestibilité ***f*** digestibility

digestif -ive ***adj*** digestive

trouble ***m*** **digestif** digestive disorder

tube ***m*** **digestif** alimentary canal

digestion ***f*** digestion

digital(e) ***adj*** digital

digitaline ***f*** digitalin (pharmaceutical properties of foxglove used for certain heart condition)

dilatateur ***m*** dilator (muscle)

dilatation ***f*** dilation; dilatation

dilatation ***f*** **des bronches** bronchial tube dilation

dilatation ***f*** **de la rate** distended spleen

dilater ***v*** to dilate

diphtérie ***f*** diphtheria

diplopie ***f*** double vision

discal(e) ***adj*** of a spinal disc

hernie ***f*** **discale** slipped disc

discarthrose ***f*** wearing away of the invertebrate disc

discret -ète ***adj*** not serious

dislocation ***f*** dislocation

disloquer ***v*** to dislocate

dispositif *m* intra-utérin (DIU) intra-uterine (contraceptive) device (IUD)
disque *m* intervertébral invertebrate disc
dissection *f* aortique aorta (main artery) rupture
dissolvant *m* nail varnish remover; solvent
distome *m* fluke (parasitic flatworm)
diurétique *m* diuretic
diurétique *adj* diuretic
diverticule *m* diverticulum (abnormal tube in alimentary tract)
diverticulite *f* diverticulitis (inflammation of a diverticulum)
diverticulose *f* colique abnormal cavities in the large intestine
DMLA (see dégénérescence)
DMP (dossier *m* médical personnel) personal medical records
docteur *m* doctor
doigt *m* finger
doigt de pied *m* toe
doigtier *m* fingerstall (cover to protect a finger)
doléance *f* complaint
dolichocôlon *m* elongation of the large intestine (not an illness)
don *m* d'organes donation of organs
don *m* du sang blood donation
donneur *m* –euse *f* donor
dopamine *f* dopamine (compound in nervous tissue)
doppler *m* pulsé ultrasound device used esp. in heart tests
doppler, vélicométrie *f* ultrasound measurement of blood-flow speed in the blood vessels
doppler *m*, echo (graphie) *f* test combining ultrasound scan and ultrasound measurement of blood-flow speed
dorsal(e) *adj* dorsal
déformation *f* dorsale back deformation
dosarthrose *f* back rheumatism
dos *m* back
  mal de dos *m* backache
  dos rond *m* (avoir le) to be round-shouldered

dosage ***m*** dosage; amount; correct proportion

dose ***f*** dose

dose ***f*** **mortelle** lethal dose

douche ***f*** **vaginale** vaginal douche

douleur ***f*** ache; pain

douleur ***f*** **aiguë** acute/sharp pain

douleurs ***fpl*** **de l'accouchement** labour pains

douleur ***f*** **colique** colic

douleur ***f*** **intermittente** intermittent pain

douleur ***f*** **irritante** nagging pain

douleur ***f*** **lancinante** throbbing pain

douleur ***f*** **persistante** constant pain

douleurs ***fpl*** **rhumatismales** rheumatic pains

douleur ***f*** **sourde** dull pain

douloureux -euse ***adj*** aching; painful

douve ***f*** fluke (parasitic flatworm)

dragée ***f*** sugar-coated pill

drain ***m*** drainage tube

drainage ***m*** drainage

drainage ***m*** **lymphatique** lymphatic

drainer ***v*** to drain

drip feeding ***m*** drip feeding

drip transfusion ***f*** drip transfusion

drogue ***f*** drug

drogue ***f*** **dure/douce** hard/soft drug

drogué(e) ***m/f and adj*** drug addict

duodénal(e) ***adj*** duodenal

ulcère ***m*** **du duodénum** duodenal ulcer

duodénite ***f*** inflammation of the duodenum

duodénum ***m*** duodenum

durcisseur ***m*** **d'ongles** nail hardener

dure-mère ***f*** dura mater (outermost membrane around the brain and spinal cord)

durillon ***m*** callus; hard skin

dysarthrie ***f*** speech disorder

dysenterie ***f*** dysentery

dysfonctionnement ***m*** dysfunction

dys(hy)idrose ***f*** eczetamous disease affecting feet and hands

dyslexie ***f*** dyslexia

dyslexique ***adj*** dyslexic
dyslipidémie/dyslipémie ***f*** abnormal fat level in the blood
dysménorrhée ***f*** dysmenorrhoea (painful or difficult menstruation)
dyspepsie ***f*** dyspepsia; indigestion
dysphagie ***f*** difficulty in swallowing
dysphasie ***f*** dysphasia (speech disorder)
dysplasie ***f*** dysplasia (abnormal tissue growth)
dysplasie ***f*** **du col de l'utérus** early cancerous growth in the cervix
dyspnée ***f*** dyspnoea (laboured breathing)
dyspnéique ***adj*** of a person who has difficulty in breathing
dystocie ***f*** (condition of) difficulty in childbirth/delivery
dystocique ***adj*** type of childbirth/delivery which is difficult
dystrophie ***f*** dystrophy
dystrophie ***f*** **musculaire** muscular dystrophy
dysurie ***f*** dysuria (painful/ difficult urination)

eau ***f*** water
eau ***f*** **dentifrice** mouthwash
eau ***f*** **gazeuse** sparkling (mineral) water
eau ***f*** **minérale** mineral water
eau ***f*** **oxygénée** hydrogen peroxide
eau ***f*** **non-potable** non-drinking water
eau ***f*** **potable** drinking water (fountains etc.)
eau ***f*** **du robinet** tap water
eau ***f*** **savonneuse** soapy water
eau ***f*** **de Seltz** seltzer; soda water
eau ***f*** **de source** spring water
eau ***f*** **thermale** thermal water
elle a perdu ***v*** **les eaux** her waters have broken
ébauche ***f*** early signs; early stages (of illness)
éblouissement, avoir ***v*** **un** to have a dizzy spell
ébouillanter ***v*** to scald
s'ébouillanter to scald oneself
écarteur ***m*** retractor (muscle)

ECG *m* (électrocardiogramme) electrocardiogram (record of heart's electrical activity)

ECBU (see examen cytobactériologique des urines)

ecchymose *f* bruise

ecchymotique *adj* bruised

masque *m* ecchymotique blotchy face (due to breathing difficulty)

écharde *f* splinter

écharpe *f* sling (arm)

échauffement *m* inflammation; overheating (of blood)

échauffement *m* du ventre constipation

échauffer *v* to overheat

échocardiographie *f* echocardiography (ultrasound heart scan)

échographe *m* ultrasound scanner

échographie *f* ultrasound scan; image produced by an ultrasound scan

échographier *v* to scan ultrasonically

écho *m*/échographie *f* ultrasound scan

écho *m* 2D 2D ultrasound scan

écho *m* 3D/échotomographie *f* 3D ultrasound scan

éclampsie *f* eclampsia; convulsions

éclater *v* to burst (blister, blood vessel, etc.)

vaisseau *m* éclaté burst blood vessel

éclisse *f* splint

éclisser *v* to put in splints

écorchure *f* abrasion

écouler *v* to seep/ooze out

écran *m* solaire sun screen (cream)

écran *m* total total sunblock (cream/lotion)

édulcorant *m* sweetener

édulcorant *m* de synthèse artificial sweetener

eczéma *m* eczema

eczéma *m* de contact eczema following (allergy-producing) contact

eczéma *m* atopique babies' eczema

eczématiforme *adj* resembling eczema

effets ***mpl*** **secondaires** side effects

efficacité ***f*** **thérapeutique** therapeutic effectiveness

éjaculation ***f*** **rétrograde** retrograde ejaculation (into bladder)

effleurage ***m*** light form of massage

effleurer ***v*** to touch/massage lightly

élancement ***m*** shooting/sharp pain

électrocardiogramme ***m*** **(**see **ECG)**

électrocardiographe ***m*** electrocardiograph (instrument which records heart's electrical activity)

électrocardiographie ***f*** examination of heart's electrical activity (electrocardiogram)

électrocution ***f*** electrocution

électrodes ***fpl*** **pour les douleurs** pain-relieving clip-on electrodes

électroencéphalogramme ***m*** electroencephalogram (record of brain's electrical activity)

électroencéphalographe ***m*** electroencephalograph (examination of brain's electrical activity)

électrolytes ***fpl*** electrolytes

électromyogramme ***m*** **(EMG)** examination of muscles' electrical activity

électrothérapie ***f*** electrotherapy

ELISA (enzyme-linked immunosorbent assay) biological test for hepatitis or AIDS virus

élimination ***f*** elimination

éliminer ***v*** to eliminate

élongation ***f*** strained/pulled (muscle)

émail ***m*** enamel (tooth)

embarras ***m*** upset

embarras ***m*** **gastrique** upset stomach

embarrasser ***v*** **l'estomac** o lie heavy on the stomach

embolie ***f*** embolism (blood clot or air bubble blockage)

embolie ***f*** **artérielle** arterial embolism

embolie ***f*** **cérébrale** cerebral embolism

embolie *f* gazeuse air embolism
embolie *f* pulmonaire pulmonary embolism
embouts *mpl* (jetables) de seringues (single-use) syringe tips
embrocation *f* embrocation
embryologie *f* embryology
embryon *m* embryo
à l'état *m* d'embryon in an embryonic condition
embryon *m* congelé frozen embryo
embryonnaire *adj* embryonic
émétique *m* emetic (medicine which causes vomiting)
éminence *f* protuberance
émollient *m* demulcent; soothing agent
émollient(e) *adj* soothing
emphysème *m* emphysema (lung condition causing breathlessness)
empirique *adj* empiric
remède *m* empirique empiric remedy
emplâtre *m* plaster
emplâtre *m* pour les cors corn plaster
empoisonnement *m* poisoning
empoisonnement *m* du sang blood poisoning
émulsion *f* emulsion (medicinal)
empreinte *f* digitale fingerprint
empreinte *f* génétique genetic fingerprint
enceinte *adj* pregnant
enceinte *f* de jumeaux -elles pregnant with twins
encéphale *m* encephalon (brain and top of spinal cord)
encéphalite *f* encephalitis (inflammation of the brain)
encéphalogramme *m* encephalogram (X-ray of the brain)
endémique *adj* endemic
endocarde *m* endocardium (inner wall of the heart)
endocardite *f* inflammation of the endocardium
endocrinologie *f* endocrinology
glandes *fpl* endocrines endocrine glands (ovaries, testicules, thyroid etc.)
endogène *adj* endogenous (originating from body interior)

endomètre ***m*** endometrium (membrane lining the uterus)

endométrite ***f*** endometritis (inflammation of the uterus lining)

endométrose ***f*** endometriosis

endoprothèse ***f*** prosthesis placed inside the body

endorphine ***f*** endorphine (morphine-like substance produced by brain)

endoscope ***m*** endoscope (instrument for internal examinations)

endoscopie ***f*** endoscopy examination

enfant ***m*** **'bleu'** 'blue' baby (baby with congenital heart or blood circulation condition)

enfant(e) ***m/f*** **mort-né(e)** still-born baby

enfler ***v*** to swell; to swell up

enflure ***f*** swelling

enfoncement ***m*** **de la boîte crânienne** fractured skull

enfoncement ***m*** **de la cage thoracique** crushed ribs

engelure ***f*** chilblain

engendrer ***v*** to bring about (an illness)

engorgement ***m*** engorgement; obstruction

engorger ***v*** to engorge; to obstruct

engourdissement ***m*** numbness

enlever ***v*** to remove (surgically)

enraidissement ***m*** stiffening or blockage (of muscle)

ensellure ***f*** saddle-shaped (normal) curvature of the spine

entérite ***f*** enteritis (inflammation of the small intestine)

entérobactérie ***f*** enterobacteria (digestive tract bacteria)

entérocolite ***f*** enterocolitis (inflammation of large and small intestines)

entérovirus ***m*** enterovirus (intestinal virus which can spread elsewhere)

enthésiopathie ***f*** tendinitis (inflammation of tendon)

entorse ***f*** sprain

entorse ***f*** **grave** serious sprain (causing torn ligaments)

entorse ***f*** **au poignet** sprained wrist

entre deux âges ***adj*** middle-aged

énurésie ***f*****, also known as 'pipi au lit'** involuntary bed wetting
enzyme ***f/m*** enzyme (biological substance aiding/allowing chemical reaction)
épanchement ***m*** effusion (abnormal presence of liquid)
épanchement ***m*** **de synovie** water on the knee
épaule ***f*** shoulder
épaule ***f*** **bloquée** blocked/ frozen shoulder
épicondyle ***m*** epicondyle (elbow joint)
épicondylite ***f*** tennis elbow
épidémie ***f*** epidemic
 seuil ***m*** **épidémique** epidemic threshold
épiderme ***m*** epidermis (outer layer of skin)
épididyme ***m*** epididymis (duct behind the testicles)
épididymite ***f*** inflammation of the epididymis
épigastre ***m*** middle of the stomach area
 douleur ***f*** **épigastrique** pain in the middle of the stomach
épiglotte ***f*** epiglottis
épilation ***f*** epilation; removal of hair
épilepsie ***f*** epilepsy
épilepsie ***f*** **généralisée** severe epilepsy
épileptique ***m/f and adj*** epileptic
état ***m*** **de mal épileptique** successive epileptic fits
épiler ***v*** to epilate; to remove hair from
épine ***f*** **dorsale** backbone
épingle ***f*** **de sûreté** safety pin
épiphyse ***f*** rounded ends of long bones
épiphysite ***f*** growing pains (child development)
épisiotomie ***f*** episiotomy (surgical cut into vagina to aid childbirth)
épistaxis ***f*** epistaxis (nosebleeding)
épithélioma; épithéliome ***m*** epithelioma (malignant tumour of epithelial tissue)
épithélium ***m*** epithelium (body surface, digestive tract and other cavity tissue)
éponge ***f*** sponge
épreuve ***f*** test; trial

épreuve *f* **d'effort démaquillée** electrocardiogram during an effort test on patient who no longer takes any medicines

épreuve *f* **de tolérance au glucose** glucose tolerance test

épuisement *m* exhaustion

grand état *m* **d'époisement** (utterly) exhausted state

épuisement *m* **dû à la chaleur** heat exhaustion

épuration *f* purification

épuration *f* **extrarénale** dialysis

éraflure *f* scratch; graze

ergonomique *adj* ergonomic

ergothérapie *f* occupational therapy (manual work)

ergothérapeute *m/f* occupational therapist

érosion *f* abrasion; erosion (of joints)

érosif -ive *adj* progressively destroys (relating to illness/ disease)

éructation *f* burp

éruption *f* rash; eruption (tooth growth through the gums)

érysipèle *m* erysipelas (reddish skin infection)

érythème *m* erythema (abnormal redness of the skin)

érythème *m* **fessier** nappy rash

érythrocyte *m* red corpuscle

érythrodermie *f* **bulleuse** serious skin allergy, manifesting redness and blisters

érythromycine *f* antibiotic

escarre *f* bedsore

Escherichia coli *m* Escherichia coli (E. coli)

esquille *f* bone splinter

essai *m* **clinique** human experiment for new drug

essentiel –ielle *adj* relating to illnesses with no known cause

estomac *m* stomach

état *m* **critique sévère** serious critical condition

étanche *adj* waterproof

éternuement *m* sneeze; sneezing

éternuer *v* to sneeze

ethmoïde *m* ethmoid (bone above nose and behind forehead)

ethmoïdite *f* sinusitis infection with inflammation of the ethmoid

étiologie ***f*** etiology/aetiology (study of causes of disease)

étiquetage ***m*** marking (products); labelling

étouffement ***m*** asphyxiation; suffocation; choking; breathlessness

étourdissement ***m*** dizzy spell; fit of giddiness

étrier ***m*** stapes (small stirrup-shaped ear bone)

euthanasie ***f*** euthanasia

eupnéïque ***adj*** of a person who breathes well

eupnéïque ***f*** medicine which aids breathing

évacuation ***f*** evacuation (draining of liquid); transport of person in accident to hospital

évacuer ***v*** to evacuate/discharge (from body)

évanoui(e) ***adj*** unconscious

(s')évanouir ***v*** to faint

évanouissement ***m*** fainting fit/spell; blackout

éveinage ***m*** vein removal

éventration ***f*** rupture

évoluer ***v*** to evolve; to develop (of illness)

évolution ***f*** development; evolution

évolutivité ***f*** progressive/worsening nature (of illness)

exacerbation ***f*** exacerbation

examen ***m*** **cardiaque** heart examination

examen ***m*** **clinique** clinical examination

examen ***m*** **complémentaire** complementary examination

examen cytobactériologique des urines (ECBU) ***m*** cytobacteriological examination

examen ***m*** **endocervical** cervical screening

examens ***mpl*** **en externe** outpatient examinations

examen ***m*** **exocervical** examination of the exterior of the cervix

examen ***m*** **du fond d'oeil** funduscopy (examination of back of the eye)

examen ***m*** **de la vue** sight test

examen ***m*** **du sang** blood test/analysis

examen ***m*** **fonctionnel** physical examination

examen *m* médical/de santé medical/ health examination
examen *m* prénuptial pre-marital examination (for marriage settlement contracts)
examen *m* radiographique X-ray or other radiation examination
examen *m* radiologique radiological examination
examiner *v* to examine
exanthème *m* redness of the skin
excentration *f* joint displacement (from centre)
excentration *f* de la rotule displaced kneecap
excipient *m* flavouring for medicine
exciter *v* to excite; to stimulate
exclu(e) *adj* used to qualify a faintly discernible organ on X-rays : a sign that the organ no longer functions
excrétion *f* excretion
excroissance *f* outgrowth
exérèse *f* surgical removal of tumour, stone, diseased organ, etc.
exophtalmie *f* abnormally globular eyes (exophthalmia)
exostose *f* bone formation (abnormal) on top of normally developed bone
expectorant *m and adj* expectorant
  intervention *f* exploratrice exploratory operation
exploration *f* exploration; detailed examination
exploratoire *adj* exploratory
extenseur *m* extensor muscle; chest expandor
extension *f* stretching (muscle, etc.); traction (limb, etc.)
externe *adj* external; exterior
  médicament *m* à usage externe medication for external use
extraction *f* extraction
extraire *v* to extract; to pull out
extrasystole *f* extrasystole (irregular heartbeat)

FA (see fibrillation auriculaire)
face *f* face
facial(e) *adj* facial
  nerf *m* facial facial nerve

paralysie *f* faciale facial paralysis

faciès *m* features

facteur *m* factor (as in protection factors for sun lotion)

facteur *m* déclenchant catalyst

facteur *m* de la coagulation blood coagulation agent

facteur *m* Rhésus Rhesus/RH factor

faible *adj* weak; feeble

faiblesse *m* mentale mental deficiency

fantasme *m* fantasy; delusion

fatigue *f* fatigue

fatigué(e) *adj* tired; weary; strained

cerveau *m* fatigué overworked brain

cœur *m* fatigué strained/overworked/weak heart

estomac *m* fatigué stomach upset

fatiguer *v* to get tired: to tire

fausse couche *f* miscarriage

fausses dents *fpl* false teeth

fausse route *f* wrong way (of food/drink going down the 'wrong way')

fauteuil *m* électrique (avec releveur) electric relaxation armchair with help-you-up function

fauteuil *m* de repos manuel manually-operated relaxation armchair/lounger

fauteuil *m* roulant wheelchair

fauteuil *m* à dossier inclinable wheelchair with reclining back

fébricule *f* light fever; slight temperature

fébrifuge *m* febrifuge; antipyretic drug or agent, e.g. cooling drink

fébrifuge *adj* febrifuge; antipyretic (preventing/reducing fever)

fébrile *adj* feverish

aplasie *f* fébrile blood disease, possibly leukaemia, with corpuscle deficiency and fever

fécondation *f* fertilisation

fecondation *f* in vitro (FIV) in vitro fertilisation

fécondité *f* fertility

fémur *m* femur

fenouil *m* fennel (plant)

fer *m* iron

ferment ***m*** **lactique** starter/ fermentation culture
fertilité ***f*** fertility
fesse ***f*** buttock
fessier -ière ***adj*** of, concerning the buttock(s)
muscles ***mpl*** **fessiers** gluteal (buttock) muscles
feuille ***f*** **de température** temperature chart
fibrillation ***f*** fibrillation (quivering movement, especially of heart muscle)
fibrillation ***f*** **auriculaire (FA)** auricular fibrillation
fibrillation ***f*** **ventriculaire** ventricular fibrillation
fibrinolise ***f*** blood clot elimination with an enzyme
fibrome ***m*** **de l'utérus** fibroid in the uterus
fibroscope ***m*** fibrescope (optic fibres instrument enabling internal examinations)
fibroscopie ***f*** fibrescope examination
fibrose ***f*** **kystique** cystic fibrosis (hereditary disease usually leading to respiratory infection)
fièvre ***f*** fever; high temperature
fièvre ***f*** **cérébrale** brain fever
fièvre de Lassa ***f*** Lassa fever (acute tropical disease)
fièvre ***f*** **ganglionnaire/ glandulaire** glandular fever
fièvre ***f*** **hémorragique** haemorrhagic fever
fièvre ***f*** **quartaine** acute fever, recurring every four days
fièvre ***f*** **jaune/typhoïde** yellow/ typhoid fever
fièvre ***f*** **paludéenne** malarial fever
fièvre ***f*** **paratyphoïde** paratyphoid fever
fièvre ***f*** **puerpérale** puerperal fever (post-natal fever caused by uterine infection)
fiévreux -euse ***adj*** feverish
fil ***m*** **dentaire** dental floss
filiforme ***adj*** long and slender (of body shape)
filtres ***mpl*** **nasaux** nosecaps
fistule ***f*** fistula (abnormal passage between organs)
fixateur ***m*** **externe** metal brace for broken bone
flacon ***m*** small bottle; phial; flask

flacon ***m*** **doseur** small bottle with measure for drops
flamber ***v*** to sterilise with a flame
flatulence ***f*** flatulence
flatuosité ***f*** flatus; wind
fléchir ***v*** to flex
fléchisseur ***m*** flexor muscle
flessum ***m*****/flexum** ***m*** blocked/ paralysed joints in flexed position
flore ***f*** **intestinale** intestinal flora
flore ***f*** **vaginale** vaginal flora (not abnormal)
fluence ***f*** **verbale** verbal fluency
fluidifiants ***mpl*** **bronchiques** cough mixtures (to release fluid in bronchial tubes)
fluor ***m*** fluorine
fluoration ***f*** fluoridation (of water, helping to preserve teeth)
fluorure ***m*** fluoride
flush ***m*** flush
flutter ***m*** excessively fast heartbeat (over 150 a minute)
flux ***m*** **sanguin** blood flow
flux ***m*** **menstruel** menstrual flow
fluxion ***f*** swelling; inflammation
fluxion ***f*** **dentaire** gumboil
fluxion ***f*** **de poitrine** pneumonia
fœtus ***m*** foetus
foie ***m*** liver
  abcès ***m*** **du foie** abcess of the liver
  cancer ***m*** **du foie** cancer of the liver
folie ***f*** lunacy; insanity; madness
follicule ***m*** follicle
follicule ***m*** **pileux** hair root cavity/gland
follicule ***m*** **ovarique** ovarian follicle
folliculite ***f*** inflammation of follicle
fonctionnement ***m*** working; functioning
fontanelle ***f*** fontanelle (boneless part of a baby's head)
forceps ***m*** forceps
forme ***f*** **pharmaceutique** pharmaceutical form (including packaging)
forme ***f*** **physique** fitness
  sous forme ***f*** **de comprimés** in tablet form

formication ***f*****/fourmillement** ***m*** pins and needles

formule ***f*** **sanguine** blood corpuscles' distribution

fosse ***f*** cavity or hollow in the body

fouler ***v*** to sprain; to twist

cheville ***f*** **foulée** sprained ankle

(se) fouler ***v*** **le poignet** to twist/sprain one's ankle

fou ***m*** **folle** ***f and adj*** crazy

foyer ***m*** **de l'infection** source of the infection

fracture ***f*** fracture

fracture ***f*** **en bois vert** single/ clean fracture

fracture ***f*** **compliquée** compound facture

fracture ***f*** **du crâne** fracture of the skull

fracture ***f*** **de fatigue** fracture due to excessive physical activity

fracture ***f*** **fermée** simple fracture; closed fracture

fractures ***fpl*** **multiples** multiple fractures

fracture ***f*** **ouverte** compound fracture; open fracture

fracturer ***v*** to fracture

fraise ***f*** strawberry mark; birthmark

fréquence ***f*** **cardiaque** heartbeat rate; pulse rate

fréquence ***f*** **respiratoire** breathing rate

frictions ***fpl*** **localisées** localised frictional massage

frisson ***m*** chill; shiver

frissonner ***v*** to shiver

froissement ***m*** strain

froisser ***v*** to strain (a muscle)

front ***m*** forehead

(os) frontal ***m*** forehead (bone)

frottement ***m*** **péricardique** abnormal rubbing noise of heartbeat

frottement ***m*** **pleural** abnormal rubbing noise with each breath (possible symptom of pleurisy)

frottis ***m*** **sanguin** blood smear

frottis cervico-vaginal ***m*** **(FCV)** cervical smear

fumigateur ***m*** fumigator

furoncle ***m*** boil; furuncle

gale ***f*** scabies; itch

galénique ***adj*** galenic (of medicine produced from animal or vegetable tissue)

galop *m*, bruit de abnormal heartbeat noise
gammagraphie *f* medical imagery using gamma rays
ganglion *m* ganglion (nerve cluster/nucleus)
ganglions *mpl*, avoir des to have swollen glands
ganglion *m* lymphatique lymph gland/node
ganglionnaire *adj* of, concerning glands
  aire *f* ganglionnaire body area containing glands (neck, armpits, groin)
gangrène *f* gangrene
gant de crêpe *m* crepe glove (used for body scrub)
gant de crin *m* massage glove
gants *mpl* latex latex gloves
garde-malade *m/f* home nurse
gargarisme *m* gargle
  (se) faire *v* un gargarisme to gargle
garrot *m* tourniquet
gastrectomie *f* gastrectomy (surgical removal of whole/part of stomach)
gastric *adj* gastric
gastrite *f* gastritis (inflammation of stomach lining)
gastroentérite *f* gastroenteritis (inflammation of stomach and intestines)
gastroentérite *f* virale gastritis due to a virus
gastroentérologie *f* gastroenterology
gastroentérologue *m* gastroenterologist (digestion specialist)
gaz *mpl* du sang different air components in the blood
gelée *f* royale royal jelly (vitamin product)
gélule *f* gelatine capsule
gelure *f* frostbite
gencives *fpl* gums
généraliser *v* to generalise
  cancer *m* généralisé cancer throughout the whole body
  infection *f* généralisée systemic infection (throughout the whole body)
(se) généraliser *v* to spread
génétique *f* genetics
  conseil *m* génétique genetic advice/information given

to future parents based on hereditary illnesses

genévrier ***m*** juniper

génie ***m*** **génétique** genetic engineering

génome ***m*** genome

génotype ***m*** genotype (genetic constitution of a person)

gentiane ***f*** gentian (gentian violet dye is used as antiseptic)

genou ***m*** knee

genouillère ***f*** knee support

genoux cagneux ***mpl*** knock-kneed

gerçure ***f*** crack; chapping

mains ***fpl*****/genoux** ***mpl*****, pleines/pleins de gerçures** badly chapped hands/knees

gériatrie ***f*** geriatry

gériatrique ***adj*** geriatric

germe ***m*** germ; first stages of organ growth

germes ***mpl*** **de blé** wheatgerm

gérontologie ***f*** gerontology

gérontopsychiatre ***m/f*** psychiatrist for the elderly

gestation ***f*** gestation; pregnancy

GEU (see grossesse extra-utérine)

GEV (see gastroentérite virale)

gibbosité ***f*** hump

gingival(e) ***adj*** gingival

pâte ***f*** **gingivale** gum ointment

gingivite ***f*** gingivitis

ginseng ***m*** ginseng (root powder)

glaire ***f*** mucus; phlegm

glaire ***f*** **cervicale** cervical mucus

glande ***f*** gland

glande ***f*** **endocrine** endocrine gland

glande ***f*** **pituitaire** pituitary gland (at base of brain)

glande ***f*** **sébacée** sebaceous gland

glande ***f*** **sudoripare** sweat gland

glande ***f*** **surrénale** adrenal gland (which secrets adrenaline)

glande ***f*** **thyroïde** thyroid gland

glandes ***fpl*** **digestives** digestive glands

glandes ***fpl*** **lacrymales** lachrymatory (tear) glands

glandes ***fpl*** **mammaires** mammary glands

glandes *fpl* salivaires salivary glands

glandulaire *adj* glandular

glaucome *m* glaucoma (diminishing eyesight)

gliome *m* brain or nerve tumour

globe *m* oculaire eyeball

globe *m* vésical shape of swollen bladder

globule *m* rouge/blanc red/ white corpuscle

globule *m* sanguin blood cell; blood corpuscle

glotte *f* glottis (upper end of windpipe)

glucose *m* glucose

glucide *m* carbohydrate

glucidique *adj* carbohydrate

index *m* glucidique sugar-in-the-blood scale related to foods

équivalence *f* glucidique sugar-count equivalence between different quantities of different foods

gluten *m* gluten (protein present in cereal grains)

glycémie *f* glycaemia (glucose level in the blood)

équilibre *m* glycémique normal and stable amounts of different glucoses in the blood

glycérine *f* /glycérol *m* glycerine /glycerol (used as laxative)

goitre *m* goitre (neck swelling)

gommage *m* du corps/du visage body/facial scrub

gomme *f* gumma (internal tissue swelling)

gomme adragante *f* tracaganth (white/reddish pharmaceutical gum dye)

gonade *f* gonad (ovary or testicle)

gonadotrophine *f* gonadotropin (substance stimulating gonads to produce sperm/egg)

gonalgie *f* gonalgy (pain in the knee)

gonarthrose *f* rheumatism of the knee

gonflement *m* swelling; (stomach) distension

gonfler *v* to swell up; to become puffy

yeux *mpl* gonflés puffy eyes

gonorrhée *f* gonorrhoea

gorge *f* throat

mal à la gorge, avoir ***v*** to have a sore throat

gourme ***f*** impetigo (contagious skin infection)

goût ***m*** taste

goutte ***f*** gout

goutte ***f*** drop (of liquid)

goutte-à-goutte ***m*** drip (feed)

goutte ***f*** **au nez** dripping/runny nose

alimenter ***v*** **au goutte-à-goutte** to put (someone) on a drip

gouttes ***fpl*** **pour le nez** nose drops

gouttes ***fpl*** **pour les oreilles** ear drops

gouttes ***fpl*** **pour les yeux** eye drops

gouttière ***f*** plaster cast; groove in bone

gouttière ***f*** **sagittale** sagittal suture (bone junction on top of skull)

grain ***m*** pellet; small pill

grain ***m*** **de beauté** beauty spot; mole

grand(e) malade ***m/f*** severely ill patient

granulome ***m*** fleshy growth on a healing cut

grave ***adj*** serious

gravelle ***f*** gravel (stones in urinary tract)

greffe ***f*** transplant; graft

greffe ***f*** **du coeur** heart transplant

greffe ***f*** **de moelle osseuse** bone marrow transplant

greffe ***f*** **d'organe(s)** organ transplant

greffe ***f*** **de peau** skin graft

greffe ***f*** **de rein** kidney transplant

greffer ***v*** to transplant; to graft

grêle ***m*** small intestine

grêle ***adj*** long and slender (of finger)

grelotter ***v*** to shiver

grésillement ***m*** crackling noise

griffe ***f*** **du diable** devil's claw

gril ***m*** **costal** rib cage

grippal(e) ***adj*** influenzal

affectation ***f*** **grippale** influenza; flu

médicament ***m*** **pour état grippal** anti-flu drug

grippe ***f*** flu

grippe ***f*** **asiatique** Asian flu

grippe ***f*** **aviaire** avian flu
grippe ***f*** **intestinale** gastric flu
grossesse ***f*** pregnancy
grossesse ***f*** **à haut-risque** high-risk pregnancy
grossesse ***f*** **extra-utérine** ectopic pregnancy
grossesse ***f*** **nerveuse** phantom pregnancy
  test ***m*** **de grossesse** pregnancy test
grosseur ***m*** lump; tumour
grossir ***v*** to put on weight; to get bigger
groupe ***m*** **sanguin** blood group/type
groupe ***m*** **tissulaire** tissue group/type
guérir ***v*** to cure; to heal
guérison ***f*** cure; healing; recovery
guérissable ***adj*** curable
gueule ***f*** **de bois** hangover
gustatif -ive ***adj*** gustative
gymnastique ***f*** **aquatique; aquagym** aquagym
gymnastique ***f*** **corrective** remedial gymnastics
gymnastique ***f*** **oculaire** eye exercises
gymnastique ***f*** **orthopédique** orthopaedic exercises
gymnastique ***f*** **respiratoire** breathing exercises
gymnastique ***f*** **suédoise** callisthenics (body work-out)
gynécologie ***f*** gynaecology
gynécologue ***m/f*** gynaecologist

haleine ***f*** breath
  mauvaise haleine ***f*** bad breath
halitose ***f*** halitosis (bad breath)
hallucination ***f*** hallucination
hallucination ***f*** **auditive** auditory hallucination
hallucination ***f*** **olfactive** olfactory hallucination
hallucination ***f*** **visuelle** visual hallucination
halluciné(e) ***m/f*** hallucinated person; lunatic
hallucinogène ***adj*** hallucinogenic; mind-expanding; 'mind-blowing' (of drug)
hallux valgus ***m*** pigeon-toed condition
hamamélis ***m*** witch-hazel
hammam ***m*** steam bath
hanche ***f*** hip

pose ***f*** **d'une prothèse de hanche** hip replacement operation
handicap ***m*** handicap; disability
handicapé(e) ***m/f*** disabled person
handicapé(e) ***adj*** disabled; handicapped
haptonomie ***f*** communication with foetus through sensory stimulation
HAV (see hépatite)
HBV (see hépatite)
HCV (see hépatite)
héliothérapie ***f*** heliotherapy (sunlight treatment)
hématie ***f*** red corpuscle
hématique ***adj*** type of liquid produced after blood coagulation
kyste ***m*** **hématique** pocket of blood resulting from a bruise
hématologie ***f*** haematology (study of blood physiology)
hématologique ***adj*** haematological
hématologue ***m/f*** haematologist (blood specialist)
hématome ***m*** bruise/haematoma
hémi- ***prefix*** semi- (meaning one side of)
hémiplégie ***f*** hemiplegia (paralysis of one side of the body)
hémiplégique ***m/f*** hemiplegic (person paralysed down one side)
hémiplégique ***adj*** hemiplegic (paralysed down one side)
hémochromatose ***f*** disease caused by excess iron in organism
hémodialyse ***f*** haemodialysis/kidney or renal dialysis
hémoglobine ***f*** haemoglobin (red oxygen-carrying protein in blood)
hémogramme ***f*** (see **formule sanguine)**
hémolyse ***f*** **pathologique** pathological haemolysis (abnormal elimination of red corpuscles)
hémolyse ***f*** **physiologique** physiological haemolysis (natural elimination of red corpuscles)
hémophile ***m/f*** haemophiliac
hémophile ***adj*** haemophiliac

hémophilie ***f*** haemophilia (hereditary condition with failure of normal blood coagulation)
hémorragie ***f*** **externe** external haemorrhage/bleeding
hémorragie ***f*** **interne** internal haemorrhage
hémorragique ***adj*** haemorrhagic
hémorroïdes ***fpl*** haemorrhoids; piles
hémorroïdal(e) ***adj*** haemorrhoidal
hémostase ***f*** haemostasis (stopping of haemorrhage)
héparine ***f*** heparin (anticoagulant in various tissues and organs)
hépatique ***m/f*** liver complaint sufferer
hépatique ***adj*** relating to the liver
hépatite ***f*** hepatitis
HAV (abbreviation **virus** ***m*** **de l'hépatite A)** hepatitis A
HBV (abbreviation **virus** ***m*** **de l'hépatite B)** hepatitis B
HCV (abbreviation **virus** ***m*** **de l'hépatite C)** hepatitis C
hépatite ***f*** **virale** viral hepatitis
hépatologue ***m/f*** liver specialist
hépatopathie ***f*** liver complaint
herbe ***f*** **médicinale** medicinal herb
héréditaire ***adj*** hereditary
hérédité ***f*** heredity
hernie ***f*** hernia; rupture
hernie ***f*** **discale** slipped disc
hernie ***f*** **étranglée** strangulated hernia (blocking circulation)
hernie ***f*** **hiatale** hiatus hernia (between chest & abdomen)
hernie ***f*** **inguinale** inguinal hernia (of the groin)
herpès ***m*** herpes
herpès ***m*** **buccal** cold sore
herpès ***m*** **circiné** ringworm
herpès ***m*** **de la lèvre** cold sore
herpès ***m*** **genital** genital herpes
herpès ***m*** **zoster** shingles
hétérogène ***adj*** suspicious aspect of organs on X-rays, scanner results, etc.
hibernation ***f*** **artificielle** induced hypothermia
hippocampe ***m*** hippocampus (ridges at the bottom of the brain's lateral ventricles)

hippocratisme *m* digital nail deformation

hirsutisme *m* hirsutism (excessive hair growth)

histamine *f* histamine (body catalyst from allergies)

histologie *f* histology (study of tissues)

HIV (abbr. of human immunodeficency virus) HIV virus

Hodgkin, maladie *f* de Hodgkin's disease

holistique *adj* holistic (of treatment taking into account mental and social factors)

holter *m* rhythmique heart activity record over a 24 hour period

homéopathie *f* homeopathy

homéopathique *adj* homeopathic

doses *fpl* homéopathiques small (therapeutic) doses

homogène *adj* homogeneous aspect of healthy organs on X-rays, scanner results, etc.

hoquet *m* hiccup; hiccough

hoqueter *v* to hiccup; to hiccough

horaire *f* nocturne nocturnal (of fever, symptoms, etc.)

hormone *f* hormone

traitement *m* hormonal treatment using hormones

trouble *m* hormonal hormone-producing glands disorder

hormonothérapie *f* course of treatment using hormones

humérus *m* humerus (upper arm bone)

huile *f* essentielle essential oil (used in medicines)

huile *f* de foie de morue cod-liver oil

huile *f* de massage massage oil

huile *f* de ricin castor oil

humeur *f* mood; humour

humeur *f* aqueuse aqueous humour/body (clear fluid in eye between the lens and cornea)

humeur *f* vitreuse vitreous humour/body (clear tissue behind eyeball lens)

hydarthrose *f* du genou water on the knee

hydratant(e) *adj* moisturising

hydratation *f* hydration

hydrate *m* de chloral chloral hydrate (sedative)

hydrater *v* to moisturise

(s') hydrater to hydrate oneself

hydrocéphalie *f* hydrocephalus (excessive fluid in the brain)

hydrocortisone *f* hydrocortisone (steroid hormone for treating inflammations/rheumatism)

hydrocution *f* immersion syncope

hydronéphrose *f* hydronephosis (water-swollen kidney)

hydropisie *f* dropsy (excess fluid in body tissues or cavities)

hydrosadénite *f* inflammation of sweat glands

hydrothérapie *f* hydrotherapy

hygiène *f* hygiene

hygiène *f* alimentaire food hygiene

hygiène *f* bucco-dentaire oral hygiene

hygiène *f* corporelle personal hygiene

hygiène *f* du travail work hygiene; hygiene at work

hygiène *f* de vie, pour une meilleure for a healthier life

hygiénisme *m* cleanliness (for good health)

hygroma *m* bursitis (inflammation of a bursa/fluid filled sac)

hymen *m* hymen

hyperactif -ive *adj* hyperactive

hyperacanthose *f* excessive growth of layer of skin

hypercholestérolémie *f* abnormal amount of cholesterol in blood

hyperdense *adj* relating to (abnormal) opacity of organ on X-rays, etc.

hyperglycémie *f* hyperglycaemia (glucose excess in blood stream)

épreuve *f* d'hyperglycémie provoquée glucose tolerance test

hyperhidrose *f* hyperhidrosis; excessive sweating

hyperkératose *f* corn (hard skin)

hypermétropie *f* long-sightedness

hyperparathyroïdie *f* hyperpathyroidism (abnormal

functioning of gland near the thyroid)

hyperphagie *f* obsessional eating (overeating)

hyperprotidique *adj* protein enriched

hypersomnie *f* prolonged sleeping; frequent sleeping

hypertensif -ive *adj* hypertensive

hypertension *f* hypertension

hypertension *f* **artérielle** high blood pressure

hypertension *f* **intracrânienne** intracranial pressure

hyperthermie *f* hyperthermia

hypertonique *adj* hypertonic (of high-tension muscles); of extremely concentrated medicine for injection **perfusion** *f* **hypertonique** hypertonic drip

hypertrophie *f* hypertrophy (organ/tissue enlargement due to increase in size of cells)

hyperventilation *f* hyperventilation (abnormally fast breathing rate)

hypnose *f* hypnosis

hypnothérapie *f* hypnotherapy

hypnotique *m* hypnotic; sleep inducing (pill)

hypnotique *adj* hypnotic

hypoallergénique *adj* hypoallergenic (of little/ reduced tendency to cause allergic reaction)

hypocondriaque *m/f* hypochondriac

hypocondriaque *adj* hypochondriac

hypocondrie *f* hypochondria

hypoglycémie *f* hypoglycaemia (glucose deficiency in bloodstream)

hypophyse *f* pituitary gland (small ductless gland at base of brain)

hypopnée *f* breathing insufficiency

hypotensif -ive *adj* hypotensive

hypotension *f* **artérielle** low blood pressure

hypothalamus *m* hypothalamus (brain area controlling hunger, thirst, temperature, etc.)

hypothermie *f* hypothermia

hypothyroïdie *f* hypothyroidism (subnormal activity of thyroid gland)

hypotrophie *m* insufficient natural growth development (due to malnutrition)
hystérectomie *f* hysterectomy
hystérie *f* hysteria
hystérographie *f* hysterography; X-ray of the womb
hystérique *m/f* hysterical person
hystérique *adj* hysterical

IAD (see insémination artificielle avec doneur)
ictère *m* jaundice; icterus
idiotie *f* idiocy
iléite *f* ileitis (inflammation of last portion of the intestine)
iléite *f* régionale Crohn's disease; regional enteritis
iléon *m* ileum (last portion of small intestine)
iliaque *adj* iliac (of the lower body or *ilium* area)
os *m* iliaque hip bone
imagerie *f* médicale medical imagery
imagerie *f* échographique ultrasound scans
imagerie *f* radiographique 2D X-rays
imagerie *f* remnographique 3D MRIs
imagerie *f* scanographique scans
imagerie *f* tomographique 3D sectional scans
imagerie par résonance magnétique nucléaire (IRM) nuclear magnetic resonance imaging (MRI)
imbécile *m/f* imbecile
imbécile *adj* imbecilic
imbécillité *f* imbecility; idiocy
immunisation *f* immunisation
immunité *f* immunity
immunité *f* acquise acquired/developed immunity
immunité *f* cellulaire cell-mediated immunity
immunité *f* naturelle inborn immunity
impaction *f* impaction (bone parts driven or wedged together and not moveable)
impuissance *f* impotence
imputable *adj* attributable to
impétigo *m* impetigo (contagious skin infection)
implant *m* implant
implant *m* capillaire hair graft

incubation ***f*** incubation
incurable ***m/f*** person that cannot be cured
incurable ***adj*** incurable
malade ***m/f*** **incurable** incurably ill
indemne ***adj*** unharmed
index ***m*** index finger; forefinger index
indication ***f*** indication
indication ***f*** **thérapeutique** remedial indication
indice ***m*** **d'Apgar** Apgar index (newborn baby's vitality rating)
IMC ***m*** **(indice de masse corporelle)** BMI (body mass index) (index which determine categories of weight; obtained by dividing body weight in kilograms by the square of the body's height in metres. Categories of body weight and their relative index figures follow)
maigreur ***f*** thinness: below 18
normal ***adj*** normal: between 18 and 25
surpoids ***m*** overweight: between 25 and 30
obésité ***f*** obesity: between 30 and 40
obésité ***f*** **massive** massively obese: result over 40
indice ***m*** **de protection solaire** sun protection factor (on bottles, tubes etc.)
indigestion ***f*** indigestion
indolore ***adj*** painless
infarctus ***m*** infarction (dead tissue through lack of blood)
infarctus ***m*** **du myocarde** heart attack; coronary thrombosis
infarctus ***m*** **pulmonaire** partial lung collapse following embolism
infarctus ***m*** **septal** heart attack affecting the ventricular septum
infecter ***v*** to infect
(s') infecter ***v*** to become infected/septic
infecté(e) ***adj*** infected
infectieux -euse ***adj*** infectious
infection ***f*** infection
infertilité ***f*** infertility
infestation ***f*** infestation
infester ***v*** to infest
infiltrat ***m*** abnormal dark spot on X-ray image

infiltration ***f*** injection; seepage; infiltration

infiltration ***f*** **graisseuse** fatty tissue build-up

infirme ***adj*** physically disabled

infirmerie ***f*** infirmary

infirmier ***m*** **-ière** ***f*** nurse

infirmier ***m*** **-ière** ***f*** **chef** charge nurse

infirmier ***m*** **-ière** ***f*** **diplômé(e) (d'état)** (state) registered nurse

infirmier ***m*** **-ière** ***f*** **libéral(e)** self-employed nurse

infirmier ***m*** **-ière** ***f*** **en -chef** head nurse

infirmier -ière major ***m/f*** (military) matron

infirmier ***m*** **-ière** ***f*** **visiteur -euse** visiting/district nurse

infirmité ***f*** infirmity

inflammation ***f*** inflammation

inflammatoire ***adj*** inflammatory

influx ***m*** **nerveux** nerve impulse

infra-rouge ***adj*** infrared

inhalateur ***m*** inhaler

inhalateur ***m*** **buccal** mouth inhaler

inhalateur ***m*** **de poche** pocket-sized inhaler

inhalation ***f*** inhalation

faire ***v*** **des inhalations** to use steam inhalations

inhaler ***v*** to inhale; to breathe in

inhibiteur ***m*** inhibitor (natural substance or medicine)

inhibiteur ***m*** **calcique** calcium blocker (treats high blood pressure)

inhibiteur ***m*** **de la coagulation** inhibitor of blood coagulation

inhibiteur ***m*** **de la pompe à protons** stomach ulcer medicine

inhibiteur -trice ***adj*** inhibitory

injecté(e) ***adj*** injected

yeux ***mpl*** **injectés de sang** bloodshot eyes

injection ***f*** injection

injection ***f*** **déchaînante** overdose (a mistakenly administered injection with potential fatal results, shortly after a previous injection with the same product)

injection ***f*** **d'insuline** insulin injection

injection *f* **intradermique** intradermic injection
injection *f* **intramusculaire** intramuscular injection
injection *f* **intraveineuse** intravenous injection
injection *f* **sous-cutanée** subcutaneous injection
inoculation *f* inoculation (injection of microbes)
inoculation *f* **accidentelle** accidental infection (through injury)
inoculer *v* to inoculate
insémination *f* **artificielle** artificial insemination
insémination *f* **artificielle avec donneur** *m* **(IAD)** artificial insemination by donor (AID)
insolation *f* sunstroke
insomniaque *m/f* insomniac
insomniaque *adj* insomniac
insomnie *f* insomnia
inspiration *f* breathing in
dyspnée *f* **inspiratoire** breathing-in difficulty
instabilité *f* **gléno-humérale** fragile/easily dislocated shoulder
instable *adj* unstable (condition)
instaurer *v* to start (course of treatment)
instillation *f* instillation (with drops for eye, ear, etc.)
institutionnaliser *v* to institutionalise (patient)
s'institutionnaliser *v* to become institutionalised
insuffisance *f* insufficiency; inadequacy (of an organ or set of organs to function properly which can lead to total failure)
insuffisance *adj* **cardiaque/rénale** cardiac/renal insufficiency
insuffisance *f* **respiratoire** respiratory insufficiency
insufflation *f* insufflation
insuffler *v* to insufflate (blow/breathe powder, gas, air into body cavity)
insuline *f* insulin
insulinodépendant(e) *adj* insulin-dependent (of person or illness)
insulinorequérant(e) *adj* requiring insulin temporarily (of person or illness)

traitement *m* par insuline insulin treatment
interaction *f* médicamenteuse adverse interaction of two medicines
intercarpien(ne) ***adj*** of/concerning the wrist bones
intercure *f* pause between two courses of treatment; temporary pause in a treatment
interféron *m* humain interferon (proteins released by cells)
interligne *f* space between two bones (used in X-ray readings)
intermission *f* intermission
intermittence *f* remittance; (heart/pulse) irregularity
interne *m/f* des hôpitaux house doctor
interne ***adj*** internal; interior
médecine *f* interne study of internal illnesses
internement *m* confinement
interner *v* to confine (someone to a mental hospital/institution)
interrompre *v* to interrupt; to terminate
interruption *f* voluntaire de grossesse (IVG) voluntary termination of pregnancy; abortion
intervenir *v* to intervene; to operate
intervention *f* intervention; operation
intervention *f* chirurgicale surgical operation
intestin *m* intestine
intestins *mpl* bowels
intestin grêle *m* small intestine; bowel
intestin gros *m* large intestine
intoxication *f* poisoning
intoxication *f* alimentaire/ toxi-infection *f* alimentaire food poisoning
intoxiqué(e) ***adj*** addicted
toxicomane *m/f* drug addict
intoxiquer *v* to intoxicate
intra- (prefix) inside; into
dermo-réaction *f* allergy testing injection (under the skin)
musculaire *m and f* intramuscular
veineux -euse ***adj*** intravenous
intubation *f* intubation
intuber *v* to intubate
invalide *m/f* disabled person

grand invalide *m* civil severely disabled person
invalide ***adj*** disabled
invasif -ive ***adj*** invasive/ spreading (disease and procedure)
investigation ***f*** examination
involution ***f*** involution (reduction in size of an organ)
iode ***m*** iodine
ionogramme ***m*** blood test to show ion count
IRM (see imagerie par résonance magnétique)
iridologie ***f*** iridology (diagnosis by examination of iris)
iris ***m*** iris
iritis ***f*** iritis (inflammation of the iris)
irradiant(e) ***adj*** radiant; spreading (pain, illness)
irradiation ***f*** irradiation
irréductible ***adj*** irreducible (of fractures, hernias)
irrégulier -ière ***adj*** anomalous; irregular
irrigateur ***m*** irrigator (hydrotherapeutic appliance to eliminate toxins in the intestines, vagina, etc)
irrigation ***f*** irrigation
irriguer ***v*** to irrigate
irritant ***m*** irritant
irritant(e) ***adj*** irritant
irritation ***f*** irritation
ischémie ***f*** ischaemia (blood circulation blockage or disorder in an organ)
isolement ***m*** isolation
isotonique ***adj*** isotonic
solution *f* isotonique solution equal in molecular concentration to blood plasma
IV (abbreviation of **intraveineux -euse)**

jambe ***f*** leg
jambe *f* de bois wooden leg
jambe *f* artificielle artificial leg
jambe *f* articulée articulated leg
jambes arquées ***fpl*** bow-legged
jarret ***m*** back of the knee
jarrets *mpl* d'acier strong legs
jaunisse ***f*** jaundice
jéjunum ***m*** jejunum (second part of small intestine)
à jeun ***adv*** on an empty stomach (required before many blood tests)

jeûne ***m*** fasting; abstention from food

jeûner ***v*** to fast

jonction ***f*** place on/in body between two organs or parts of organs

jonction ***f*** **atrio-ventriculaire/ auriculo-ventriculaire** heart area between the auricles and ventricules

joue ***f*** cheek

'ses jours ***mpl*** **ne sont pas en danger'** 'no mortal danger' bulletin (for a patient)

jumeau ***m*** **-elle** ***f*** twin

jumeaux ***mpl*** **-elles** ***fpl*** twins

jumeaux ***mpl*** triceps sural (the two calf muscles)

kaliémie ***f*** potassium level in the blood

Kaposi, maladie ***f*** **de/sarcome** ***m*** **de/syndrome** ***m*** **de** Kaposi's illness/sarcoma/syndrome (malignant tumour syndrome)

kératine ***f*** keratin (fibrous proteins in hair)

kératite ***f*** keratitis (inflammation of the cornea)

kératose ***f*** keratosis (thickening of the cornea)

kératoplastie ***f*** cornea graft

kiné(e) ***m/f*** **(abbr. of kinésithérapeute)** physio (physiotherapist)

kinésithérapeute ***m/f*** physiotherapist; physical therapist

kinésithérapie ***f*** physiotherapy

kleptomanie ***f*** kleptomania

kyste ***m*** cyst

kyste ***m*** **de l'ovaire** ovarian cyst

kyste ***m*** **sébacé** sebacious (fatty) cyst

kystique ***adj*** cystic

L-dopa ***f*** L-dopa (form of dopa: a treatment for Parkinson's disease)

lésion ***f*** **kystique** cystic lesion; cyst (internal)

labial(e) ***adj*** labial

labile ***adj*** unstable (products); changing (mood, condition)

laboratoire ***m*** laboratory

laboratoire ***m*** **d'analyses médicales** medical analysis laboratory

laboratoire *m* biochimique biochemical laboratory

laboratoire *m* de virologie virology laboratory

laboratoire *m* pathologique pathological laboratory

laboratoire *m* physiologique physiological laboratory

laboratoire *m* radiochimique radiochemical laboratory

lacération *f* laceration

lacrymal(e) -aux *adj* lachrymal (relating to tears)

liquide *m* lacrymal; larmes *fpl* tears

glande *f* lacrymale lachrymal gland

lactation *f* lactation

lactobacilles *mpl* lactobacilli (bacteria producing lactic acid)

lactose *m* lactose (sugar in milk)

lait *m* milk; lotion

lait *m* pour le corps body lotion

lait *m* de croissance vitamin-enriched milk

lait *m* cru unpasteurised milk

lait *m* maternisé baby milk formula

lait *f* de toilette cleansing lotion; cleansing milk

lait *f* de toilette pour bébé baby lotion

lame *f* drop (of liquid)

lame *f* criblée flat bone between brain and nose

lampe *f* de luminothérapie avec écran de protection light therapy lamp with protective screen

lancette *f* lancet (surgical knife)

langue *f* tongue

langue *f* blanche/chargée/pâteuse coated or furred tongue

lanoline *f* lanoline

laparotomie *f* laparotomy (stomach operation)

laparotomie *f* exploratrice investigative laparotomy

laryngectomie *f* laryngectomy (removal of part or entire larynx)

laryngite *f* laryngitis

laryngoscope *m* laryngoscope (instrument)

laryngoscopie *f* laryngoscopy (detailed inspection of larynx using a laryngoscope)

larynx ***m*** larynx

laser ***m*** laser

lassitude ***f*** lassitude

latéralisation ***f*** natural tendency to be right- or left-handed/ footed

lavage ***m*** washing

lavage ***m*** **gastrique** stomach wash

lavage ***m*** **interne** douche

lavage ***m*** **intestinal** intestinal wash

lavement ***m*** enema; fluid or syringe used for enema

lavement ***m*** **à la Gastrograffine ®** ***f*** iodine base enema fluid (used in preparation for scanning the large intestine)

lavement ***m*** **barité** barium enema (pre X-rays: coloscopy more usual)

laver ***v*** to wash

laxatif ***m*** laxative

laxatif -ive ***adj*** laxative

légionellose ***f*** (see **maladie du légionnaire)**

lentigo ***m*** mole; lentigo

lentilles ***fpl*** **de contact** contact lenses

lèpre ***f*** leprosy

léser ***v*** to damage; to injure

lésé(e) ***adj*** damaged

lésion ***f*** lesion

lésion ***f*** **pulmonaire** pulmonary lesion

lésion ***f*** **cérébrale** brain damage

lésions ***fpl*** **internes** internal injuries

létal(e) ***adj*** lethal

léthargie ***f*** lethargy

leucémie ***f*** leukaemia

leucocyte ***m*****; globule** ***m*** **blanc** white corpuscle

leucoplasie ***f*** leucoplasy (abnormal white patch/blotch on tongue/inside mouth/on genitals)

leucorrhée ***f*** leuc(k)orrhea (vaginal discharge)

leucotomie ***f*** leucotomy (surgery to white nerve fibres in the brain)

lèvre ***f*** lip

lèvre ***f*** **supérieure/inférieure** upper/lower lip

lèvres ***fpl*** **d'une incision/d'une plaie** edges of an incision/a wound

libérer ***v*** to unblock

libido ***f*** libido

licenciement ***m*** discharge (of patient)

lifting ***m*** facelift

ligament ***m*** ligament

ligature ***f*** ligature (esp. in surgery)

ligaturer ***v*** to ligature; to tie up; to bind

light ***adj*** diet (of drinks)

limaçon ***m*** **osseux** cochlea (snail-shaped cavity inside the ear)

lime ***f*** **à ongles** nail file

lingettes ***fpl*** baby wipes

lingual(e) ***adj*** related to the tongue

protraction ***f*** **linguale** putting out the tongue

linguette ***f*** tablet taken under the tongue

lipase ***f*** lipase (fat-breaking enzyme)

lipasémie ***f*** amount of lipase in the blood

lipide ***m*** lipid; fatty acid/oil/wax/ steroid

lipomatose ***f*** presence of fatty cysts; increase in body fat under the skin

lipome ***m*** fatty cyst

liposoluble ***adj*** liposoluble (fat-soluble)

liposuccion ***f*** liposuction

lipping ***m*** osteophyte (abnormal shape/extension to bone on edge of rheumatic joint)

liquide ***m*** **amniotique** amniotic fluid

liquide ***m*** **synovial** synovial fluid/liquid (lubricates joints and tendon sheathes)

listériose ***f*** listeriosis (food-poisoning infection)

lit ***m*** bed

lit ***m*** **d'eau** water bed

lit ***m*** **privé** private bed (hospital room)

lithiase ***f*** lithiasis (kidney stones causing inflammation)

lithiase ***f*** **rénale** lithiasis (kidney stones causing inflammation)

lithiase ***f*** **urinaire** gravel (crystals formed in urinary tract)

lobe ***m*** **de l'oreille** ear lobe

lobe ***m*** **inférieur/moyen/ supérieur** lower/middle/upper lobe (of lung)

lobotomie *f* **cérébrale** lobotomy (pre-frontal brain lobe incision)

local *m* **d'examens** examination room

lombaire *adj* lumbar

lombalgie *f* lumbago

longévité *f* longevity

lordose *f* lordosis (inward curvature of the spine)

lotion *f* lotion

lotion *f* **après-soleil** after-sun lotion

lotion *f* **calmante à la calamine** calamine lotion

lotion *f* **capillaire** hair care lotion

lotion *f* **contre les insectes** insect repellant

loucher *v* to squint

loupe *f* fatty cyst; wen (benign skin tumour); magnifying glass

lucite *f* skin disease/burn from too much sunlight

luette *f* uvula (fleshy extension of soft palate hanging above throat)

lumbago *m* lumbago

luminothérapie *f* light therapy

lunettes *fpl* glasses

lunettes *fpl* **bifocales** bifocal spectacles

lunettes *fpl* **de glacier** snow glasses

lunettes *fpl* **de natation** swimming goggles

lunettes *fpl* **noires** dark glasses

lunettes *fpl* **de plongée** diving goggles

lunettes *fpl* **de protection** safety goggles

lunettes *fpl* **de sécurité** safety glasses

lunettes *fpl* **de soleil** sunglasses

lunettes *fpl* **de vue** corrective vision glasses

lupus *m* lupus (ulcerous skin disease)

lupus *m* **érythémateux disséminé** systemic lupus erythematosis (lupus infection throughout the body)

lupus *m* **éryhthémateux chronique** chronic lupus erythematis

lupus *m* **vulgaire** lupus vulgaris (TB with dark red skin patches due to TB inoculation)

luxation *f* dislocation

luxer *v* to dislocate

lymphangite ***f*** lymphangitis (inflammation of lymphatic vessels)

lymphatique ***adj*** lymphatic

système ***m*** **lymphatique** lymphatic system (network of vessels conveying lymph)

lymphe ***f*** lymph (colourless fluid with only white corpuscles)

lymphosarcome ***m*** lymphosarcoma (cancer of the lymph gland/node tissue)

lyse ***f*** lysis (cell/bacteria destruction)

lytique ***adj*** relating to/causing lysis

cocktail ***m*** **lytique** possibly lethal combination of medicines, would cause lysis through a cell-destroying (lytic) process

mâchoire ***f*** **inférieure/supérieure** lower/upper jaw

mâchonnement ***m*** bruxism (grinding or clenching of teeth); chewing

mâchonner ***v*** to chew

macrobiotique ***adj*** macrobiotic (Zen Buddhist dietary system)

macrobiotique ***f*** macrobiotics

macrocytose ***m*** abnormally large red corpuscles

macroscopique ***adj*** macroscopic (visible to the naked eye)

macula ***f*** macula (spot-like central area of retina)

macule ***f*** macula (dark spot in the skin)

magnésium ***m*** magnesium

magnétisme ***m*;** magnetism (for rheumatism, lumbago, kidney stones, etc.)

magnétothérapie ***f*** magnetism

maigre ***adj*** underweight; thin

maigrir ***v*** to slim

main ***f*** hand

maïeuticien ***m*** (rarely used word) male mid-wife

maison ***f*** **de retraite médicalisée** nursing home

majeur ***m*** middle finger

majoration ***f*** increase (in); rise (in)

majorer ***v*** to increase (dose, etc.)

mal ***m*** **à la gorge** sore throat

mal ***m*** **à l'estomac** stomach ache

mal au cœur, avoir ***v*** to feel ill/sick

mal au cœur en voiture, avoir ***v*** to feel carsick

mal ***m*** **aux dents** toothache

mal ***m*** **aux oreilles** earache

mal ***m*** **aux reins** backache

mal ***m*** **de dents** toothache

mal ***m*** **de dos** backache

mal ***m*** **des montagnes** mountain sickness

mal ***m*** **de mer** seasickness

mal ***m*** **de tête** headache

mal ***m*** **des transports** travel sickness

mal partout, avoir ***v*** to ache all over

malade ***m/f*** invalid; patient; sick person

malade ***m/f*** **ambulatoire** ambulatory patient

malade ***m/f*** **imaginaire** hypochondriac

malade ***m/f*** **mental(e)** mentally ill/mentally sick person

faux -sse malade ***m/f*** malingerer

grand(e) malade ***m/f*** seriously ill person

malade ***adj*** ill

gravement malade ***adj*** gravely/seriously ill

maladie ***f*** illness; disease

maladie ***f*** **d'Addison** Addison's disease (progressive anaemia, weakness and bronzing discolouration of skin)

maladie ***f*** **d'Alzheimer** Alzheimer's disease

maladie ***f*** **aiguë** short, violent illness

maladie ***f*** **aiguë de l'appareil respiratoire** acute respiratory disease

maladie ***f*** **à virus Ebola** Ebola virus/disease

maladie ***f*** **de Basedow** Basedow's disease (excessive hormone production following thyroid gland inflammation)

maladie ***f*** **bénigne** mild/harmless illness

maladie ***f*** **bleue** 'blue' disease; congenital cyanosis (oxygen-deficient blood)

maladie *f* **bronzée** Addison's disease (see also **maladie d'Addison**)
maladie *f* **des caissons** decompression sickness
maladie *f* **cardio-vasculaire** cardiovascular disease
maladie *f* **de/par carence** (any) deficiency disease
maladie *f* **du charbon** anthrax (biological) disease
maladie *f* **chronique** chronic disease
maladie *f* **contagieuse** contagious disease
maladie *f* **coronarienne** coronary heart disease
maladie *f* **du coeur** heart disease
maladie *f* **de Fanconi** Fanconi disease (congenital illness causing poor reproduction of red corpuscles)
maladie *f* **héréditaire** hereditary disease
maladie *f* **d'Hodgkin** Hodgkin's disease
maladie *f* **infantile** childhood disease/complaint
maladie *f* **infectieuse** infectious disease
maladie *f* **de langueur** wasting disease
maladie *f* **du légionnaire** legionnaires' disease
maladie *f* **mentale** mental illness
maladie *f* **mortelle** fatal illness/disease
maladie *f* **post-opératoire** post-operative illness
maladie *f* **de Parkinson** Parkinson's disease
maladie *f* **de peau** skin disease
maladie *f* **professionnelle** industrial disease
maladie *f* **rare** rare disease
maladie *f* **sexuellement transmissible (MST)** sexually transmitted disease (STD)
maladie *f* **du sommeil** sleeping sickness
maladie *f* **du travail** occupational disease
maladie *f* **tropicale** tropical disease
maladie *f* **vénérienne** venereal disease (VD)

malaise ***m*** feeling of sickness/ fainting
malaise ***m*** **cardiaque** mild heart attack
malaise ***m*** **vasovagal** sudden drop in blood pressure
malaria ***f*** malaria
malentendant(e) ***m/f*** person hard of hearing
malformation ***f*** abnormality
malignité ***f*** malignancy
malin -igne ***adj*** malignant (worsening/growing illness/ tumour)
malléolaire ***adj*** concerning protruding sides of ankle bone
malvoyant(e) ***m/f*** partially sighted person
mammaire ***adj*** mammary
  abcès ***m*** **mammaire** mammary abscess
  glandes ***fpl*** **mammaires** mammary glands
  hypertrophie ***f*** **mammaire** breast enlargement
  plastie ***f*** **mammaire** cosmetic breast surgery
mammectomie ***f*** mammectomy
mammographie ***f*** mammography (2D breast X-ray)
manchette ***f*** **plâtrée** wrist plaster (cast)
mandibule ***f*** mandible (jaw)
mandibulaire ***adj*** concerning the mandible
manie ***f*** mania (serious mental disorder)
manipulation ***f*** manipulation
manipulation ***f*** **vertébrale** manipulation of the spine
manipulations ***fpl*** **génétiques** genetic engineering
manuel ***m*** **de premiers soins** first-aid manual
maquillé(e) ***adj*** of treatment not stopped sufficiently in advance of examination for a true result
marasme ***m*** marasmus (emaciation due to nutritional deficiency)
marcher ***v*** **en dormant** to sleep walk
marqueur ***m*** marker (in blood tests, shows development or diminution of illness); tracer

(radioactive isotope trace in medical imagery)

marron ***m*** **d'Inde, extrait de** horse chestnut preparation

martial(e) ***adj*** concerning iron

carence ***f*** **martiale** lack of iron

masque ***m*** mask

masque ***m*** **anti-pollution** anti-pollution mask

masque ***m*** **à oxygène** oxygen mask

masque ***m*** **chirurgical** surgical mask

masque ***m*** **de grossesse** chloasma (dark patches on face occurring sometimes in pregnancy)

masque ***m*** **hydratant** moisturising face pack

masque ***m*** **respiratoire** breathing mask

massage ***m*** massage

massage ***m*** **cardiaque** cardiac massage

massage ***m*** **du cuir chevelu** scalp massage

masser ***v*** to massage

se faire masser ***v*** to have a massage

masseur -euse ***m/f*** masseur -euse

mastectomie ***f*** mastectomy

mastication ***f*** mastication; chewing

mastite ***f*** mastitis (breast inflammation)

mastoïde ***f*** mastoid process (protuberance on bone behind the ear)

mastoïde ***adj*** mastoid (conical shaped)

mastoïdite ***f*** mastoiditis (inflammation of mastoid process)

matelas ***m*** mattress

matelas ***m*** **de balnéothérapie** *f* balneotherapy mat (in the bath)

matelas ***m*** **de balnéothérapie télécommandé** remote-controlled balneotherapy mat

matières ***fpl*** **fécales** faeces

matériel ***m*** **génétique** genetic material

matériel ***m*** **métallique** metal material (nail, screw, plate, etc.) used for surgical implants

matériel ***m*** **de synthèse** synthetic material used for surgical implants

matrice *f* womb; uterus
descente de matrice *f* prolapse of the womb
maturation *f* maturation (formation of pus in abscess; cell development to maturity)
mauvaise grippe *f*, **- rougeole** *f* **etc.** serious attack or bout of flu/measles etc.
mauvaise haleine *f* bad breath
maxillaire *m* jawbone
maxillaire *adj* maxillary (concerning jawbone)
maxillaire *m* **inférieur/supérieur** lower/upper jawbone
méat *m* meatus (body channel/passage)
méat *m* **auditif** ear passage to drum
méat *m* **urinaire** urine outlet in male and female genitals
mécanicien(ne) *m/f* **dentiste** dental technician
mécanique *adj* mechanical (applied to body movements and also medical treatment apparatus)
mèche *f* pack; surgical/medical dressing
mèche *f* tent (lint/linen inserted into a wound); wick (gauze strip inserted into wound)
mécher *v* to pack (open wound) with gauze
médicaliser *v* to provide with medical care
médecin *m* doctor; physician
médecin *m* **conseil** social security/health insurance medical officers (supervising health expenditure)
médecin *m* **consultant** doctor consulted by another doctor
médecin *m* **de garde** duty doctor
médecin *m* **généraliste** general practitioner (GP)
médecin *m* **d'hôpital** consultant
médecin *m* **légiste** forensic scientist; forensic surgeon
médecin *m* **militaire** army medical officer
médecin *m* **scolaire** school doctor
médecin *m* **spécialiste** specialist

médecin *m* du travail company doctor; company doctor with own surgery or mobile unit
médecine-ball *m* medicine ball (large, heavy exercise ball)
médecine *f* medicine

list of medical specialities:
allergologie *f* allergies
anatomie *f* et cytologie *f* pathologiques pathology, anatomy and cytology (study of cells)
anesthésiologie *f* et réanimation *f* chirurgicale anaesthesiology and post-operative reanimation
cancérologie *f*, oncologie *f* médicale cancer and oncology
cardiologie *f*, affections *fpl* cardio vasculaires heart and blood-vessel conditions
chirurgie *f* générale general surgery
chirurgie *f* infantile child surgery
chirurgie *f* de la main surgery to the hand
chirurgie *f* faciale facial surgery
chirurgie *f* orthopédique orthaepedic surgery
chirurgique *f* plastique/ reconstructrice plastic/ reconstructive surgery
chirurgie *f* urologique urinary system surgery
chirurgie *f* vasculaire vascular (blood-vessel) surgery
chirurgie *f* viscérale visceral surgery (to principal body organs)
dermatologie *f* dermatology
diabétologie *f*, nutrition *f* diabetes, nutrition
échographie *f* echography (ultrasound scanning)
endocrinologie *f* et métabolisme endocrine glands and metabolism
gastroentérologie *f* et appareil *f* digestif gastroenterology (study/treatment of stomach and digestive system disorders)
gériatrie *f* geriatrics
gynécologie *f* gynaecology
imagerie *f* médicale medical imagery (X-rays, scans, etc.)
médecine *f* alternative/douce/ naturelle alternative/non-conventional/natural medicine

médecine *f* curative remedial medicine
médecine *f* légale forensic medicine
médecine *f* manuelle ostéopathie osteopathy
médecine *f* parallèle complementary medicine
médecine *f* préventive preventive medicine
nephrology *f* nephrology (kidneys)
neurologie *f* neurology
ophtalmologie *f* opthalmology
oto-rhino-larynogolgie *f* ear, nose and throat
pédiatrie *f* paediatrics
pneumologie *f* pneumology
psychiatrie *f* psychiatry
psychiatrie *f* de l'enfant et de l'adolescent child and adolescent psychiatry
radiothérapie *f* radiotherapy
rhumatologie *f* rheumatology (arthritis and rheumatism)
stomatologie *f* stomatology (mouth diseases)
vénéréologie *f* venereology

médiat(e) ***adj*** mediate (medium for obtaining result)
auscultation *f* mediate stethoscope examination
medical(e) ***adj*** medical
médicament ***m*** medicine; drug; remedy
médicament *m* allopathique conventional medicine
médicament *m* analgésique analgesic medicine
médicament *m* de confort over-the-counter pain relieving medicines (not usually reimbursed, even if prescribed)
médicament *m* contre la stérilité fertility drug
médicament *m* homéopathique homeopathic medicine/remedy
méditation *f* meditation
médullaire ***adj*** medullary (relating to the spinal cord)
compression *f* médullaire compression of spinal cord (leading to paralysis)
mégalomanie *f* megalomania
mélancolie *f* melancholia
mélancolique ***adj*** melancholic

mélanine ***f*** melanin (pigment, tanning under sun and/or UV rays)
mélanisme ***m*** melanism (excessive melanin darkening the skin)
mélanome ***m*** melanoma (tumour, usually malignant, from melanin-forming cells)
méléna/melaena ***m*** dark blood in faeces
mélilot ***m*** yellow melilot; sweet clover
mélisse ***f*** balm
membrane ***f*** membrane
membre ***m*** **supérieur/inférieur** upper/lower limb
mémoire ***f*** memory
Ménière, vertige ***m*** **de/maladie** ***f*** **de** Ménière's disease
méninge ***f*** meninx (membrane covering brain and other nervous system organs)
méningiome ***m*** meninx tumour
méningite ***f*** meningitis
méningite ***f*** **cérébro-spinale** spinal meningitis
méningocoque ***m*** meningococcus (microbe causing some forms of meningitis)
méniscal(e) ***adj*** of/concerning meniscus
lesion ***f*** **méniscale** deterioration/wasting of knee cartilage
ménisectomie ***f*** surgical removal of meniscus
ménisque ***m*** meniscus (rounded cartilage in knee)
ménopause ***f*** menopause
ménopausée ***adj*** post-menopausal
ménopausique ***adj*** menopausal
ménorragie ***f*** menorrhagia (abnormally long menstruation)
menstruation ***f*** menstruation
menstruel(le) ***adj*** menstrual
flux ***m*** **menstruel** period
menthe ***f*** **poivrée** peppermint
menton ***m*** chin
mentonnière ***f*** chin bandage
mercure ***m*** mercury
mésencéphale ***m*** midbrain; mesencephalon
mère ***f*** **porteuse** surrogate mother (illegal in france)

mesmérisme ***m;*** **magnétisme** ***m*** hypnosis (using a magnet)
mésothérapie ***f*** skin or sub-cutaneous injections
métabolisme ***m*** metabolism
métacarpe ***m*** metacarpus (hand bone)
métastase ***f*** metastasis (transfer of disease within the body)
métastaser ***v*** to metastasise (transfer disease)
métatarse ***m*** metatarsus (foot bone)
météorisme ***m*** meteorism (air-inflated stomach and intestines)
méthode ***f*** method
mettre ***v*** to apply (ointment, etc.); to put on
meurtrir ***v*** to bruise
meurtri(e) ***adj*** bruised
être ***v*** **tout meurtri** to be covered in bruises; to be black and blue all over
mg (abbreviation of **milligramme** ***m*****)** milligramme
microbe ***m*** germ; microbe
microbiologie ***f*** microbiology
microbiologiste ***m/f*** microbiologist
miction ***f*** urination
mieux-être ***m*** better general state of mental or physical well-being
migraine ***f*** migraine
mille-pertuis ***m*** St John's wort (for infusions)
mince ***adj*** slim; slender
minceur ***f*** slimness; slenderness
régime ***m*** **minceur** slimming diet
minéralité ***f*** calcium level in bones
minerve ***f*** surgical collar
minipilule ***f*** minipill
minoxidil ***m*** minoxidil (drug causing dilatation of blood vessels)
mise en garde ***f*** warning
ml (abbreviation of **millilitre** ***m*****)** millilitre
mm3 (abbreviation of **millimètre cube)** cubic millimetre
mnésique ***adj*** of/concerning to the memory
mode ***m*** **d'administration** instructions (for taking medicine/pills)

mode ***m*** **d'emploi** directions for use (medicines)
moelle ***f*** marrow; medulla
moelle ***f*** **osseuse** bone marrow
moignon ***m*** stump (of limb)
molaire ***f*** molar (tooth)
mollet ***m*** calf
moniliase ***f*** moniliasis; candidosis; thrush (white patchy infection of the mouth and throat and/or the vagina)
moniteur ***m*** **cardiaque** heart-rate monitor
monitorage; monitoring ***m*** monitoring
mononucléose ***m*** **infectieuse** glandular fever
monstruosité ***f*** deformity
monte-escaliers ***m*** stairlift
morphine ***f*** morphine
morphologie ***f*** morphology (general aspect/form of body/organs)
morsure ***f*** bite
morsure ***f*** **venimeuse** venomous bite
mort ***f*** death
mort ***m/f*** deceased person
mort ***f*** **cérébrale** brain death
mort ***f*** **clinique** clinical death (by observation of patient's condition)
mort ***f*** **naturelle** natural death
mort ***f*** **subite (inexpliquée) du nourisson** (unexplained) cot death
mort ***f*** **volontaire** suicide
trouver ***v*** **la mort** to die or be killed
morve ***f*** nasal mucus (col.); glanders (contagious disease affecting jaws and nostrils, transmitted by horses)
motricité ***f*** motivity (normal mobility of body)
mou; molle ***adj*** soft
parties ***fpl*** **molles** soft body parts (skin, muscle, nerves, intestines, etc. but not bone or cartilage)
mouche-bébé ***m*** nasal instrument for withdrawal of babies' mucus
mouchoirs ***mpl*** **en papier** paper hankies; tissues
mourir ***v*** to die
moyens ***mpl*** **thérapeutiques actuels** current methods of treatment

mucoviscidose *f* mucoviscidosis (pancreatic disease)
muguet *m* thrush (mouth and throat or vaginal infection)
multiple *adj* multiple
muqueuse *f* mucous membrane
muqueux -euse *adj* mucous
muscle *m* muscle
  biceps *m* **brachial** biceps brachii muscle (arm)
  biceps *m* **crural** biceps femoris muscle (thigh)
  grand pectoral *m* greater pectoral muscle (on chest)
  quadriceps *m* **(fémoral)** quadriceps femoris (thigh) muscle
muscles fessiers *mpl* gluteal muscles (buttocks)
musculaire *adj* muscular
musculature *f* musculature (body/organs muscular system)
mutagène *adj* mutagenic
  agent *m* **mutagène** mutagen (agent promoting genetic change)
mutisme *m* mutism (following psychological shock or mental illness)
mutité *f* dumbness; muteness
myasthénie *f* myasthenia gravis (rare chronic disease with muscular weakness)
myocardite *f* myocarditis (heart inflammation diseases)
mycologie *f* mycology (study of fungi)
mycologiste *m* fungi specialist
mycose *f* fungal disease; fungus (med.)
mycose *f* **du pied** athlete's foot
mycose *f* **vaginale** vaginal thrush
mycotoxine *f* mycotoxin (toxic substance produced by a fungus)
myélite *f* myelitis (inflammation of spinal cord)
myocarde *m* myocardium (heart muscle)
myodynie *f* muscular pain in rheumatism and cramps
myoglobine *f* myoglobin (iron-content protein in muscle cells)
myome *m* **utérin** womb-muscle tumour
myopathie *f* myopathy (progressive muscle atrophy)
myope *adj* myopic (short-sighted)

myopie ***f*** myopia; short-sightedness

myxœdème ***m*** myxoedema (thyroid disorder resulting in overweight, physical and mental lethargy)

nævus ***m*** naevus; birthmark

nævus ***m*** **simple** beauty spot or birthmark

nævus ***m*** **nævocellulaire** birthmark or beauty spot with potentially cancerous cells

nanisme ***m*** dwarfism

narcolepsie ***f*** narcolepsy (disease with fits of sleepiness)

narcose ***f*** narcosis (insensibility)

narcotique ***m*** drug; narcotic

narcotique ***adj*** narcotic

narine ***f*** nostril

nasal(e) ***adj*** nasal

natation ***f*** swimming

naturopathie ***f*****; naturothérapie** ***f*** naturopathy (natural treatment: without medicines)

nausée ***f*** nausea

nausées ***fpl*** **matinales** morning sickness

nécrose ***f*** necrosis (death of body tissue or part)

(se) nécroser ***v*** to self-destruct

la peau ***f*** **s'est nécrosée** the skin wasted away/was destroyed

négatif -ive ***adj*** negative

néoformation ***f*** new tissue formation; tumour

néonatal(e) ***adj*** neonatal

période ***f*** **néonatale** neonatal period

ne pas laisser ***v*** **à la portée** ***f*** **des enfants** ***mpl*** keep out of children's reach

néphrite ***f*** nephritis (inflammation of the kidneys); Bright's disease

néphrose ***f*** nephrosis (chronic kidney disease)

néphrologue ***m/f*** kidney specialist

néoplasme ***m*** new, abnormal tissue growth/tumour

nerf ***m*** nerve

nerf ***m*** **crural** thigh nerve

nerf ***m*** **moteur** motor nerve

nerf ***m*** **optique** optic nerve

nerf ***m*** **phrénique** phrenic nerve (relating to the diaphragm)

nerf ***m*** **pneumogastrique** pneumogastric nerve
nerf ***m*** **rachidien** spinal nerve
nerf ***m*** **sciatique** sciatic nerve
nerf ***m*** **sensitif** sensory nerve
nerf ***m*** **vague** vagus nerve
nerfs ***mpl*** **crâniens** cranial nerves
nerfs ***mpl*** **spinaux** spinal nerves
nerfs ***mpl*** **à vif (idiom)** edgy/nervy (eg. **avoir** ***v*** **les nerfs à vif** to be edgy)
avoir ***v*** **les nerfs** ***mpl*** **fragiles** to be highly strung
nerveux –euse ***adj*** nervous
grossesse ***f*** **nerveuse** phantom pregnancy; false pregnancy
système ***m*** **nerveux** nervous system
nervosité ***f*** nervousness; nervous tension
neural(e) ***adj*** neural
neurasthénie ***f*** depression; neurasthenia
neurasthénique ***m/f*** depressed person; neurasthenic
neurasthénique ***adj*** depressed; neurasthenic
neurinome ***m*** nerve tumour
neuroleptique ***m*** neuroleptic (sedative)
neuroleptique ***adj*** neuroleptic
neurologie ***f*** neurology
neurologique ***adj*** neurological
neurologue ***m*** neurologist
neuro-musculaire ***adj*** neuromuscular (concerning nerves and muscles)
neuronal(e) ***adj*** neuronal
neurone ***m*** neuron (nerve cell)
neurone ***m*** **moteur** motor neuron
neurotonique ***adj*** nervous; irritable
neutraliser ***v*** to counteract; to neutralise
névralgie ***f*** neuralgia
névralgie ***f*** **cervico-brachiale** neuralgia running from neck down the arm
névralgie ***f*** **faciale; névralgie** ***f*** **du trijumeau** short, violent pain in the face
névralgique ***adj*** neuralgic
centre/point névralgique ***m*** nerve centre
névrite ***f*** neuritis (inflammation of the nerves)
névrome ***m*** neuroma (tumour)

névrose *f* neurosis
névrose *f* **obsessionnelle/ névrose** *f* **phobique** obsessional/phobic neurosis
névrotique *adj* neurotic
nez *m* nose
nez *m* **bouché** blocked nose
NFS (see numération formule sanguine)
nicotinisme; nicotisme *m* nicotine addiction; nicotine poisoning
nodule *m* nodule (small swelling or lump)
nodus *m*; **nodosité** *f* node
noisette *f* **de gel** blob of gel
nombril *m* navel; umbilicus
noradrénaline *f* noradrenaline (hormone causing nerve or muscle impulse)
normal(e) *adj* normal
de dimension *f* **normale** normal-sized; standard-sized
nosocomial(e)*adj* nosocomial (of infectious illnesses contracted in hospitals, clinics, surgeries)
nourrisson *m* newborn baby; unweaned baby
nouveau-né(e) *m/f* new-born baby
noyade *f* drowning
mort *f* **par noyade** death by drowning
noyau *m* nucleus
nulligeste *adj* nulligest (of a woman who has never been pregnant)
numération *f* numeration
numération *f* **formule sanguine** blood count
numération *f* **globulaire** blood count
nuque *f* nape of the neck
nutritif -ive *adj* nourishing; nutritive
nutrition *f* nutrition
nutritionnel(le) *adj* nutritional
bilan *m* **nutritionnel** nutritional report (for a patient)
nystagmus *m* nystagmus (rapid, unintentional eye movements)

obèse *adj* obese
obésité *f* obesity
objectif -ive *adj* objective (of symptom which can be objectively verified/measured)

oblitérer ***v*** to obstruct
observation ***f*** observation
observation ***f*** **médicale** doctor's report
être/mettre ***v*** **en observation** to be under/to put under observation
obstétricien (ne) ***m/f*** obstetrician
obstétrique ***f*** obstetrics
obstétrique ***adj*****/obstétrical(e)** ***adj*** obstetric(al)
clinique ***f*** **obstétrique** obstetric clinic
obstruction ***f*** obstruction; blockage
obturer ***v*** to fill (teeth)
dent ***f*** **obturée** filled tooth
occipital(e) ***adj*** referring to occipital bone
région ***f*** **occipitale** occipital area (rear of the skull)
occiput ***m*** occiput (back of the head)
occlure ***v*** to occlude (block or close up pores or orifice)
occlusion ***f*** occlusion
occlusion ***f*** **intestinale** intestinal blockage
occlusion ***f*** **palpébrale** completely closed eyelid
oculiste ***m/f*** oculist; eye specialist
odontologie ***f*** odontology; dentistry
odorat ***m*** sense of smell
avoir ***v*** **l'odorat fin** to have a keen sense of smell
œdème ***m*** oedema; dropsy
œdème ***m*** **du poumon** pulmonary oedema (water-filled lungs)
œdème ***m*** **réactionnel** lump after a bump or wound
œdipe, complexe d' ***m*** Oedipus complex
œil ***m*****, yeux** ***mpl*** eye, eyes
œil ***m*** **poché; oeil au beurre noir** ***m*** black eye
avoir ***v*** **les yeux qui se croisent** to be cross-eyed
œillère ***f*** eyebath; eyecup
œsogastrectomie ***f*** oesogastrectomy (removal of part of gullet and stomach)
œsophage ***m*** oesophagus; gullet
œsophagite ***f*** inflammation of the oesophagus

œsophagite *f* **peptique** inflammation of the oesophagus

œstrogène *m* oestrogen (female hormone)

OGM (abbreviation of **organisme** *m* **génétiquement modifié)** GMO (genetically modified organism)

oignon *m* bunion

olécrâne *m* olecranon (elbow bone)

olfaction *f* olfaction; sense of smell

oligoasthénospermie *f* low sperm count

oligoélément *m* trace element (for normal growth)

oligurie *f* oliguria (reduced urination capacity)

ombilic *m* navel; umbilicus

omoplate *f* scapula (shoulder blade)

oncogène *m* oncogene (gene which can transform a cell into a tumour cell: present in tobacco smoke)

oncologie *f* oncology (study/ treatment of cancer)

oncologue *m* cancer specialist

onctueux -euse *adj* smooth; creamy

ondulant(e) *adj* uneven, irregular (pulse)

ongle *m* nail

ongle *m* **de la main** fingernail

ongle *m* **de l'orteil** toenail

ongle *m* **du pied** toenail

ongle *m* **dédoublé** split nail

ongle *m* **incarné** ingrowing nail

ongles *mpl* **cassants** fragile/ brittle nails

ongles *mpl* **soignés** well-manicured nails

onychomycose *f* onychomycosis (fungal disease affecting nails)

opacité *f* (in medical imagery) dark area(s) of organ which should normally have clear appearance

opération *f* operation

opération *f* **à cœur ouvert** open-heart surgery

opération *f* **ambulatoire** operation without overnight hospitalisation

salle *f* **d'opération** operating theatre

opéré(e) ***m/f*** patient who has been operated on

opérer ***v*** to operate

(se) faire opérer to have an operation

opiat ***m*** opiate (a sedative)

ophtalmie ***f*** ophthalmia; eye inflammation

ophtalmie ***f*** **des neiges** snow-blindness

ophtalmologie ***f*** ophthalmology

ophtalmologiste ***m/f*****; ophtalmologue** ***m/f*** ophthalmic optician; oculist; eye specialist

opticien ***m*** **-ienne** ***f*** (dispensing) optician

oral(e) ***adj*** oral

par voie ***f*** **orale** to be taken orally

oralement ***adv*** orally

orbite ***f*** eye-socket; orbit

orchite ***f*** orchitis (inflammation of the testicles)

ordinateur ***m*** **de diagnostic** diagnostic computer

ordonnance ***f*** written prescription

ordonner ***v*** to prescribe

oreille ***f*** ear

bouchon ***m*** **d'oreille (pour l'eau)** ear plug (for keeping out water)

boule ***f*** **Quiès ® (pour bruit)** ear plug (for keeping out noise)

oreille ***f*** **externe** outer ear; auricle

oreille ***f*** **interne** inner ear

oreillette ***f*** auricle

oreillette ***f*** **droite/gauche** right/left auricle

orifice ***m*** **de l'oreillette** atrium (upper heart cavity)

oreillons ***mpl*** mumps

organe ***m*** organ

organes ***mpl*** **digestifs** digestive organs

organes ***mpl*** **génitaux** genital organs

organisme ***m*** human body; organism

organisme ***m*** **génétiquement modifié (see OGM)**

orgelet ***m*** sty(e)

origan ***m*** marjoram (oil extract)

ORL (abbreviation of **oto-rhino-laryngologiste)**

orteil ***m*** toe

gros/petit ***m*** **orteil** big/little toe

orthèse ***f*** support/appliance enabling limb to function
orthodontie ***f*** orthodontics (teeth straightening)
orthopédie ***f*** orthopaedics (study and treatment of bones, joints, muscles)
orthopédique ***adj*** orthopaedic
chirurgie ***f*** **orthopédique** orthopaedic surgery
appareil ***m*** **orthopédique** orthopaedic appliance
orthophonie ***f*** speech therapy
orthopnée ***f*** inability to breathe lying down
orthoptie ***f*** eye movement therapy
orthoptiste ***m/f*** orthoptist (eye-movement therapist)
ortie ***f*** **piquante** stinging nettle
os ***m/mp*** bone
os ***m*** **du carpe** carpus (wrist bone)
os ***m*** **iliaque** hip bone
os ***m*** **de la hanche** hip bone
os ***m*** **du métacarpe** metacarpus (hand bone)
os ***m*** **pyramidal** one of small wrist bones
Osgood, maladie ***f*** **d'** Osgood's disease (leg growing pains)
osseux -euse ***adj*** bony
ossification ***f*** ossification (the process of becoming bone)
ostéite ***f*** osteitis (inflammation of bone or bone diseases)
ostéo-arthrite ***f*** osteoarthritis (degenerative disease of the joints)
ostéodensitométrie ***f*** examination measuring bone density and calcium content
ostéomalacie ***f*** osteomalacia (lack of bone calcium)
ostéome ***m*** bone tumour (harmless)
ostéomyélite ***f*** osteomyelitis (inflammation of bone or of bone marrow)
ostéopathe ***m/f*** osteopath
ostéopathie ***f*** osteopathy
ostéophyte ***m*** osteophyte
ostéoporose ***f*** osteoporosis (brittle and fragile bones)
ostéosarcome ***m*** osteosarcoma (bone cancer)
ostéosclérose ***f*** osteosclerosis (abnormal thickening of bone)

ostéosynthèse ***f*** internal fixation of a bone fracture using metal nails, screws, plates

otite ***f*** **(externe/interne)** otitis; ear infection (of outer/inner ear)

oto-rhino-laryngologie ***f*** otorhinolarynology (study and treatment of ear, nose and throat conditions)

oto-rhino-laryngologiste -gue ***m/f*** ear, nose and throat specialist

otologie ***f*** otology (study of ear diseases)

otologiste/-logue ***m/f*** otology specialist

ouate ***f*** **chirurgicale** surgical cotton wool; surgical cotton

ouate ***f*** **hydrophile** cotton wool

ouïe ***f*** hearing

avoir ***v*** **l'ouïe fine** to have a sharp sense of hearing

ovaire ***m*** ovary

overdose ***f*** overdose

ovulation ***f*** ovulation

ovule ***m*** ovum (cell)

ovule ***m*** pessary; vaginal suppository

ovuler ***v*** to ovulate

oxygène ***m*** oxygen

bouteille ***f*** **d'oxygène** oxygen cylinder/bottle

masque ***m*** **à oxygène** oxygen mask

oxygénothérapie ***f*** oxygen treatment

oxyure ***m*** pinworm; threadworm

oxyurose ***f*** enterobiasis; oxyuriasis (illness caused by pinworm/threadworm)

pacemaker ***m*** pacemaker

Paget, maladie ***f*** **cutanée de** Paget's cancer of the nipple

Paget, maladie ***f*** **osseuse de** Paget's bone deformation disease

palais ***m*** palate

palais ***m*** **fendu** cleft palate

pâleur ***f*** pallor; paleness

palliatif -ive ***adj*** palliative (pain-relieving)

palpation ***f*** palpation (medical examination, by touch)

palpébralé(e) (*pl* -aux) *adj* relating to the eyelids

réflexe ***m*** **palpébral** blinking reaction

palper *v* to palpate (examine medically by touch)

palpitant *m (informal)* ticker (heart)

palpitant(e) *adj* quivering (such as flesh); throbbing (pain)

chair *f* **palpitante** quivering flesh

palpitations *fpl* palpitations

paludéen(ne) *adj* malarial

paludisme *m* malaria

panaris *m* whitlow (inflammation next to nail)

pancréas *m* pancreas

pancréatite *f* pancreatitis (pancreas inflammation)

pancréatique *adj* pancreatic

panoramique *m* **dentaire** X-ray of all the teeth

pansement *m* dressing; bandage

pansement *m* **adhésif** adhesive plaster

pansement *m* **compressif** compressive bandage

pansement *m* **sec/humide** dry/moist dressing

pansement *m* **occlusif** hermetically sealed plaster

pansement *m* **pour ampoules** plaster for blisters

mettre *v* **un pansement** to dress (a wound)

refaire *v* **(un pansement)** to put a clean dressing on (a wound)

panser *v* to dress (wound); to put a dressing on (wound); to bandage to fill a tooth provisionally

papier *m* **hygiénique** toilet paper

papier *m* **toilette** toilet paper

papille *f* papille (small button-like protuberance of organ or body part)

papille *f* **gustative** taste bud

papille *f* **de la langue/papille** *f* **linguale** taste bud

papillome *m* papilloma (small harmless growth); wart

papillotage *m* involuntary continual blinking or eye movement

papule *f* papule or papula; pimple

papulo-pustule *f* papulo-pustule (pimple containing pus)

paracétamol *m* paracetamol

parage ***m*** cleansing of wound/ cut, removing any immediately surrounding dead skin

paralysé(e) ***m/f*** paralysed

paralyser ***v*** to paralyse

paralysie ***f*** palsy; paralysis

paralysie ***f*** **agitante** palsy, with uncontrollable tremors

paralysie ***f*** **cérébrale** cerebral palsy

paralysie ***f*** **faciale** facial paralysis

paralysie ***f*** **infantile** infantile paralysis; polyomyelitis

paramédical(e) ***adj*** paramedical

paranoïa ***f*** paranoia

paraplégie ***f*** paraplegia (paralysis of legs)

paraplégique ***m/f*** paraplegic man/woman

paraplégique ***adj*** paraplegic

parasite ***m*** parasite

parasitaire ***adj*** parasitical

parasitique ***adj*** parasitical

parathyroïde ***f*** parathyroid gland

parathyroïde ***adj*** parathyroid

paratyphoïde ***f*** paratyphoid fever

paratyphoïde ***adj*** paratyphoid

parenchyme ***m*** soft tissue part of lung, kidney and other organs

parésie ***f*** paresis; partial paralysis

paresthésie ***f*** abnormal skin sensitivity to touch or to heat

parfum ***m*** perfume/scent; flavour

pariétal(e) (pl -aux) ***adj*** parietal (concerning the wall of the body or any of its cavities) **douleur** ***f*** **pariétale** parietal pain in the chest or rib area (not the heart)

Parkinson, maladie ***f*** **de** Parkinson's disease

paroi ***f*** (anatomical) wall

parotide ***f*** saliva gland

parotidite ***f*** parotiditis (inflammation of saliva gland)

parotidite ***f*** **ourlienne** mumps

paroxysme ***m*** paroxysm (crisis point/climax)

partir ***v*** to pass on/away

parturiente ***adj*** parturient (about to give birth)

parturition ***f*** (natural) childbirth

pastille ***f*** **pour la toux** cough lozenge/drop/pastille

pastilles ***fpl*** **pour la gorge** throat pastilles

patch ***m*** **à la nicotine** nicotine patch

patch-test ***m*** patch test

pâte ***f*** cream

pâte ***f*** **dentifrice** toothpaste

pathogène ***adj*** pathogenic

agent ***m*** **pathogène** pathogen (causing disease)

pathologie ***f*** pathology

pathologique ***adj*** pathological

pathologiste ***m/f*** pathologist (disease specialist)

patient(e) ***m/f*** patient

paume ***f*** palm

paupière ***f*** eyelid

paupière ***f*** **inférieure/supérieure** lower/upper eyelid

pavillon ***m*** **auriculaire** auricle (ear)

pavillon ***m*** **de l'oreille** pinna; outer (part) ear

peau ***f*** skin

peau ***f*** **grasse/sèche** greasy/dry skin

peau ***f*** **morte** dead skin; scurf

peau ***f*** **de pêche** peach-like complexion

peau ***f*** **relâchée** loose/slack skin

pectoral ***mpl*** **(pl. -aux)** pectoral muscle

pectoral(e) ***adj*** concerning the chest; pectoral

sirop ***m*** **pectoral** cough syrup/mixture

pédalier ***m*** small hand or foot pedalling exercise machine

pédiatre ***m/f*** paediatrician

pédiatrie ***f*** paediatrics

pédiculose ***f*** pediculosis; infestation with lice

pédicure ***m/f*** chiropodist

peeling ***m*** skin peeling treatment (usually laser)

PEG (abbreviation of **polyéthylène glycol** ***m*****)**

peigne ***m*** comb

peigne ***m*** **à poux** fine-tooth comb (for removing lice)

(se) peigner ***v*** to comb (oneself)

pelade ***f*** alopecia

pellagre ***f*** pellagra (disease due to deficiency of nicotine acid)

pellicules ***fpl*** dandruff

lotion ***f*** **antipelliculaire** dandruff lotion

pelvis ***m*****;bassin** ***m*** pelvis

pénicilline ***f*** penicillin

pénis ***m*****; verge** ***f*** penis

pepsine ***f*** pepsin (enzyme in gastric juice)

peptique ***adj*** peptic (concerning or promoting digestion)

ulcère ***m*** **peptique** peptic ulcer (duodenal or stomach ulcer)

percer ***v*** to lance; to burst

percussion ***f*** percussion (body tapping as part of diagnosis); body massage

percutané(e) ***adj*** percutaneous (through the skin)

percuter ***v*** to percuss

perforation ***f*** perforation

perforer ***v*** to perforate

perfusion ***f*** drip; perfusion

perfusion ***f*** **hypertonique** drip containing an extremely concentrated liquid

mettre ***v*** **sous perfusion** to put on a drip

périarthrite ***f*** periarthritis (inflammation of ligaments and tendons surrounding a joint)

périarthrite ***f*** **scapulo-humérale** inflammation of shoulder tendons and ligaments

péricarde ***m*** pericardium (heart's membraneous sac)

péricardite ***f*** pericarditis (inflammation of the pericardium)

péridurale ***f*** epidural

péridural(e) ***adj*** epidural (relating to the outermost membrane around brain and spinal cord)

périménopause ***f*** menopause starting process

périnée ***m*** perineum (area between anus and scrotum or vulva)

période ***f*** stage (particularly of illness)

période ***f*** **d'incubation** incubation period

périodes ***fpl*** **menstruelles** periods

périodique ***adj*** recurring (illness or fever); periodic

péristaltisme ***m*** peristalsis (automatic digestive movements)

péritoine ***m*** peritoneum (serum-producing stomach membrane)

péritonite *f* peritonitis (inflammation of the peritoneum)

péritonéal(e) *adj* concerning the peritoneum

carcinose *f* **péritonéale** advanced stage of a stomach cancer which extends to the peritoneum

perlèche *f* inflammation at the corners of the lips

pernicieux -euse *adj* pernicious; ruinous

péroné *m* fibula (lower and outer leg bone)

peroxyde *m* peroxide

perruque *f* wig

perspiration *f* slight perspiration

perte *f* loss or losing

perte *f* **de connaissance** fainting; loss of consciousness

perte *f* **de mémoire** memory loss

perte *f* **de poids** weight loss

pertes *fpl* **blanches** vaginal discharge; leucorrhea

pertes *fpl* **de sang** *m* heavy bleeding

pèse-bébé *m* weighing scales for babies

pèse-personne *m* **à cadran aiguille** weighing scales with dial

pèse-personne *m* **digital** digital weighing scales

pessaire *m* pessary (womb support/contraceptive); vaginal supository

peste *f* plague

petite santé *f*, **avoir une** poor health, to be in

petite figure *f*/**mine** *f*, **avoir une** to look pale/wan

pétrir *v* to knead

pétrissage *m* kneading massage

phagocytose *f* phagocytosis (ingestion of bacteria through the white corpuscles)

phalange *f* phalanx (finger bone)

phanères *mpl* skin protectors (body and head hair, finger and toe nails)

pharmacie *f* chemist's; pharmacy

pharmacie *f* **de garde** after hours (duty) pharmacy

pharmacien(ne) *m/f* pharmacist

pharmacodépendance ***f*** drug dependency

pharmacodynamie ***f*** study of effects of medicine on the body

pharmacologie ***f*** pharmacology

pharyngite ***f*** pharyngitis (inflammation of the pharynx)

pharynx ***m*** pharynx (membrane-lined cavity behind the mouth and nose)

phase ***f*** phase; stage

phimosis ***m*** phimosis (constriction of the foreskin)

phlébite ***f*** phlebitis (inflammation of veins)

phlébologue ***f*** vein specialist

phlébolithe ***m*** calcification in a small blocked vein

phobie ***f*** phobia

phosphore ***m*** phosphorus

photophobie ***f*** photophobia (aversion to light)

photosensibilisation ***f*** photosensitisation (reaction to light)

physiologie ***f*** physiology

physiothérapeute ***m/f*** physiotherapist

physiothérapie ***f*** physiotherapy; natural medicine

phytothérapeute ***m/f*** herbalist

phytothérapie ***f*** phytotherapy (herbal medicine)

pian ***m*** yaws (contagious tropical disease)

pied ***m*** foot

pied d'athlète ***m;*** **mycose du pied** ***f*** athlete's foot

pied ***m*** **bot** club foot

avoir ***v*** **pieds plats** ***mpl*** to be flat-footed

pie-mère ***f*** pia mater (innermost membrane around brain and spinal cord)

pierre ***f*** stone

pierreux -euse ***adj*** calculous (stony)

pigment ***m*** pigment

pigmentation ***f*** pigmentation

pile ***f*** battery

pilule ***f*** pill

minipilule ***f*** minipill

pilule ***f*** **contraceptive** contraceptive pill

pilule ***f*** **abortive; pillule** ***f*** **du lendemain** abortion pill; morning-after pill

pilulier ***m*** pill box

pince ***f*** **à échardes** tweezers (for removing splinters)

pince *f* **à ongles** nail clippers
pincement *m* pinch
pincer *v* to pinch
pinçon *m* blood blister; pinch mark
'pipi *m* **au lit'; énurésie** *f* involuntary bed wetting
piquer *v* to give an injection/jab; to sting
(se) faire piquer *v* to have an injection
piquer *v* **une colère** *f* to fly into a rage
piquer *v* **une crise** *f* to throw a fit
piquer *v* **une crise** *f* **de larmes** to have a crying fit
piquer *v* **un fard** *m* to go scarlet/bright red
piquer *v* **une suée** *f* to come out in/break into a sweat
  se faire piquer to have an injection
  se piquer *v* **le doigt** to prick one's finger
piqûre *f* sting/bite (insect); injection
piqûre *f* **d'abeille/de guêpe** bee/wasp sting
piqûre *f* **d'épingle** pinprick
piqûre *f* **de méduse** jellyfish sting
piqûre *f* **de rappel** booster shot
pituitaire *adj* pituitary
pityriasis *m* pityriasis (flaking skin condition)
placebo *m* placebo
placenta *m* afterbirth; placenta
plaie *f* sore; cut; wound
planification *f* **familiale /planning** *m* **familial** family planning
plantain *m* **majeur** greater plantain (plant, used as mild laxative)
plantaire *adj* plantar (of/concerning the sole of the foot)
plante *f* **du pied** sole of the foot
  voûte *f* **plantaire** arch of the foot
plaque *f* surgical metal plate
plaque *f* **dentaire** dental plaque
plaquettes *fpl* platelets (for coagulation)
plasma *m* plasma
plasma *m* **sanguin** blood plasma
plastie *f* plastic surgery
plateau *m* horizontal part of bone

pleural(e) ***adj*** pleural (of/concerning thorax and lung membranes)
pleurésie ***f*** pleurisy
pleurétique ***adj*** pleuritic
plâtre ***m*** plaster
plâtrer to put/set in plaster
plèvre ***f*** pleura (membrane lining thorax and covering lungs)
plexus ***m*** plexus (nerve network)
plexus ***m*** **solaire** solar plexus
plombage ***m*** tooth filling
 perdre ***v*** **un plombage** to lose a filling
pneumallergène ***m*** allergy-producing particle in air
pneumoconiose ***f*** pneumoconiosis (dust-in-the-lungs disease)
pneumocoque ***m*** pneumococcus (bacteria causing pneumonia and other infections)
pneumonie ***f*** **virale** viral pneumonia
poche ***f*** sewn up part of large intestine after surgery
poche ***f*** **de glace** ***m*** ice pack
poche ***f*** **de sang** haematoma
podologie ***f*** chiropody
poids ***m*** weight
poignet ***m*** wrist
poil ***m*** body hair
poilu(e) ***adj*** hairy
poing ***m*** fist
point ***m*** point; place; spot
mise au point ***f*** development (of medicine(s))
point ***m*** **névralgique** nerve centre
point ***m*** **noir** blackhead
point ***m*** **de suture** stitch; suture
point de côté stitch (ache in the side)
point ***m*** **de compression** pressure point
pointe ***f*** tip; point
poison ***m*** poison
poitrine ***f*** chest
poliomyélite ***f*** poliomyelitis
pollakiurie ***f*** pollakiuria (frequent urination in small amounts)
pollution ***f*** pollution
pollutions ***fpl*** **nocturnes** spontaneous ejaculation during sleep (wet dreams)
polyarthrite ***f*** polyarthritis; multiple arthritis

polyarthrite *f* chronique évolutive (PCE) rheumatoid arthritis

polyarthrite *f* rhumatoïde (PR) rheumatoid arthritis

polyéthylène *m* glycol (PEG) glycerol used in small doses as a laxative

polygraphie *f* recording of several precisely measured medical tests

polyinsaturé(e) *adj* polyunsaturated (fat/oil molecule)

polymyosite *f* polymyositis (rare muscle disease)

polynévrite *f* polyneuritis (nervous disorder)

polype *m* polyp/polypus (small internal growth)

polypectomie *f* surgical removal of polyp(s)

polypnée *f* rapid breathing

polyurie *f* abnormal increase in urination amounts

polyvalent(e) *adj* polyvalent

vaccin *m* polyvalent vaccine with several different functions

pommade *f* ointment (skin); cream (hair)

pommade *f* antibiotique antibiotic ointment

pommade *f* anti-infection disinfectant

pommade *f* pour les lèvres lip salve; balm

pomme *f* d'Adam Adam's apple

pommette *f* cheekbone

pompe *f* stomacale stomach pump

pompier *m* fireman

pondéral(e) *adj* relating to body weight

ponction *f* lombaire lumbar puncture

pontage *m* bypass (operation/surgery)

pontage *m* cardiaque heart bypass operation

pontage *m* coronarien coronary bypass

poplité(e) *adj* relating to back of the knee

creux *m* poplité hollow behind the knee

porphyrie *f* porphyria (rare hereditary blood disease)

porteur *m* -euse *f* carrier (of germs, viruses, etc.)

porteur *m* sain carrier of germs, viruses, etc. but in themselves not affected

pose *f* d'un plâtre setting (of limb, bone)

poser *v* to fit (an appliance or artificial limb)

positif -ive *adj* positive

résultat *m* faux positif falsely positive result (second test advisable)

posologie *f* directions for use (medicines)

poste *m* de secours first-aid post

posthectomie *f*; circoncision *f* circumcision

post-cure *f* after-care

post-opératoire (abbrev. post-op) *adj* post-operative

post-partum *m* post-partum (period immediately following childbirth)

post-natal(e) *adj* postnatal

posttraumatique *adj* of (a) complication(s) following a physical or mental trauma

posture *f* posture

pot *m* de chambre chamber pot

pot *m* d'enfant potty

potassium *m* potassium

Pott, mal *m* de Pott's disease (TB of the spine)

pou *m* (-x *pl*) louse (lice)

pouce *f* thumb

poudre *f* powder

poudre *f* dentifrice tooth powder

poudre *f* épaississante instant thickener (for food)

pouls *m* pulse

prendre *v* le pouls to take a pulse

pouls *mpl* centraux neck or groin pulses

pouls *mpl* périphériques outer pulses (wrists, temple, etc.)

poumon *m* lung

poussée *f* dents teething

Pouteau-Colles, fracture *f* de Pouteau-Colles' (arm) fracture (lower end of the radius)

praticien(ne) *m/f* practitioner

pratiquer *v* to practise; to perform

précautions *f* d'emploi precautions before use (medicines)

précoce *adj* precocious; early (of diagnosis)

pré-éclampsie *f* pre-eclampsia (pregnancy condition)
préhension *f* gripping; prehension (ability)
prélèvement *m* sample; sampling (of blood, stools, etc.)
prélèvement *m* **de sang/de selles/d'urine** blood/stool/ urine sample
prélever *v* **un échantillon** to take a sample
prélever *v* **un organe** to remove an organ
prématuré(e) *adj* premature
premiers soins *mpl* first aid
prendre to take
prendre froid to catch cold
préopératoire *adj* preoperative
préparation *f* preparation (treatment) of patient before investigation or surgery
préparation *f* **magistrale** magistral(devised and specially made-up) medicine, on prescription
prépuce *m* foreskin
presbyacousie *f* decline in hearing (with age)
presbyacousie *f* **précoce** premature decline in hearing
presbytie *f* long-sightedness
prescription *f* verbal prescription; doctor's instructions/recommendations
prescrire *v* to prescribe
prescrit(e) *adj* prescribed
date *f* **prescrite** prescribed date
dose *f* **prescrite** prescribed dose
présentation *f* presentation (child delivery position)
présentation *f* **par la tête/par le siège** head/breech position at childbirth
préservatif (masculin) *m* condom
préservatif (feminin) *m* female condom; vaginal contraceptive device
pression *f* **artérielle** blood pressure
prévention *f* prevention
priapisme *m* priapism (persistent erection)
primaire *adj* primary (of symptoms)
prion *m* prion (proteinous infection particle: associated with Creutzfeldt-Jakob disease)
pris(e) *adj* affected; taken
gorge *f* **prise** hoarse throat

nez *m* pris stuffy nose
prise *f* de sang blood sample; the taking of a blood sample
processus *m* infectieux symptoms and consequences of infection
processus *m* cancéreux cancerous growth
processus *m* xiphoïde xiphoid process (cartilage below the sternum)
produit *m* product
produit *m* désinfectant disinfectant
produit *m* pharmaceutique pharmaceutical product
produit du confort médical medical pain-relieving product
produit *m* sanguin blood product (red corpuscles, platelets)
produit *m* bio organic product
produit *m* diététique health-food product
progestérone *f* progesterone (steroid hormone in the uterus)
prolapsus *m* prolapse (slipping forward/down of a part/organ of body)
utérin *m* (womb) prolapse
prompt(e) *adj* speedy
prompt rétablissement *m* speedy recovery
pronation *f* pronation (forearm or hand)
pronostic *m* prognosis
pronostic *m* réservé reserved prognosis
prophylaxie *f* prophylaxis (preventive treatment)
propriétés *fpl* properties (characteristics)
propriétés *fpl* thérapeutiques therapeutic properties
prostate *f* prostate gland
cancer *m* de la prostate prostate cancer
prostatectomie *f* prostatectomy (partial/total prostrate gland removal)
prostatique *adj* relating to the prostate gland
adénome *m* prostatique benign tumour of the prostate
se faire opérer *v* de la prostate to have a prostate operation
prostatite *f* prostatitis
protection *f* contre les maladies health care

protection *f* maternelle et infantile health care for mothers and young children
protège-slip *m* panty liner
(se) protéger *v* to protect oneself
protéine *f* protein
prothèse *f* prosthesis
prothèse *f* acoustique hearing aid
prothèse *f* auditive hearing aid
prothèse *f* de la hanche hip replacement
prothèse *f* mammaire breast prosthesis
prothèse *f* valvulaire artificial (heart) valve
prothrombine *f* prothrombotic substance in blood which aids coagulation
prurit *m* pruritus (severe itching)
prurit *m* anal anal pruritus (severe anal itching)
psittacose *f* psittacosis (contagious bird disease)
psoas *m* (muscle psoas-iliaque) iliopsoas muscle (one of two muscles which flex the hip joint)
psoriasis *m* psoriasis (skin condition)
psy (abbreviation for **psychanalyste, psychiatre, etc.)**
psychanalyse *f* psychoanalysis
psychanalyste *m/f* psychoanalyst
psychiatre *m/f* psychiatrist
psychiatrie *f* psychiatry
psychiatrique *adj* psychiatric
trouble *m* psychiatrique psychiatric disorder
hôpital *m* psychiatrique mental/psychiatric hospital
psychologie *f* psychology
psychologique *adj* psychological
psychologue *m/f* psychologist
psychométrique *adj* psychometric (divination quality or feature)
tests *mpl* psychométriques psychometric tests
psychopathe *m/ f* psychopath
psychopathe *adj* psychopathic
psychopathie *f* psychopathy
psychose *f* psychosis
psychose *f* maniacodépressive manic depression

psychosomatique ***adj*** psychosomatic (of physical illness caused or worsened by mental stress)
psychothérapie ***f*** psychotherapy (often abbrev. to thérapie *f*)
psychotrope ***m and adj*** sedative
puberté ***f*** puberty
pubien(ne) ***adj*** pubic
pubis ***m*** pubis
poils ***mpl*** **du pubis** pubic hair
puéricultrice ***f*** paediatric nurse in a hospital; nursery nurse
puériculture ***f*** paediatric care; infant care; nursery nursing
puerpéral -e ***adj*** puerperal (caused by childbirth)
fièvre ***f*** **puerpérale** puerperal fever (postnatal fever due to uterine infection)
pulmonaire ***adj*** pulmonary
pulpe ***f*** **dentaire** dental pulp (physiological tissue inside tooth)
pulsation ***f*** pulsation; (heart/artery) beat
pulvérisateur ***m*** spray; vaporiser
pulvérisation ***f*** spraying
pupille ***f*** pupil (eye)
purgatif ***m*** purge; purgative
purgatif -ive ***adj*** purgative
purgation ***f*** purgation; purge; purgative
purge ***f*** purge; purgative
purger ***v*** to purge
purificateur ***m*** **d'air** air steriliser
purpura ***m*** purpura (purple skin rash)
purulent(e) ***adj*** containing pus
pus ***m*** pus
pustule ***f*** pustule
pustulose ***f*** pustulosis
puvathérapie ***f*** PUVA treatment/therapy (with UV rays)
pyélite ***f*** pyelitis (inflammation of the pelvis)
pyélonéphrite ***f*** inflammation of the kidney and pelvis
pylore ***m*** pylorus (stomach opening to small intestine)
rétrécissement ***m*** **du pylore** pylorus stricture (condition in babies)
pyloroplastie ***f*** operation to widen a stricture of the pylorus

pyorrhée *f* alvéolaire pyorrhoea (shrinking of gums and loosening of teeth)

pyramidal(e) ***adj*** relating to spinal cord nervous system

syndrome ***m*** **pyramidal** paralysis of half the body

pyrogène ***adj*** pyrogenic (producing body heat or fever)

pyrosis ***m*** pyrosis (gastric acid return in the throat)

QI (abbreviation of **quotient intellectuel)** IQ (see below)

quadriceps ***m*** **(fémoral)** (femoral) quadriceps (the four-headed thigh muscle)

quadriplégie ***f*** quadriplegia (paralysis of all four limbs)

quarantaine ***f*** quarantine

mettre ***v*** **en quarantaine** to quarantine; to put into quarantine

quarantenaire ***adj*** quarantine

quatrième âge ***m*** over-75 age group

queue ***f*** **de cheval** 'pony tail' nerve cluster at end of spinal cord

syndrome ***m*** **de la queue de cheval** symptoms caused by crushed nerve cluster at end of spinal cord

queue ***f*** **du pancréas** end of the pancreas

Quick, temps ***m*** **de** blood test measuring rate of coagulation

quinine ***f*** quinine

Quinke, œdème ***m*** **de** oedematous allergic reaction (with swollen face and possibly the throat)

quinte ***f*** **de toux** coughing fit

quotient ***m*** **intellectuel** intelligence quotient (IQ)

rachialgie ***f*** rachialgy (spinal column pain)

rachis ***m*** rachis (spinal/vertebral column)

rachitique ***adj*** rachitic; concerning a rickets sufferer

être ***v*** **rachitique** to have rickets

rachitisme ***m*** rickets; rachitis

racine ***f*** **dentaire** tooth root

racine ***f*** **nerveuse** nerve root

racler ***v*** to scrape

se racler ***v*** **la gorge** to clear one's throat

radial(e) ***adj*** of/concerning radius bone

artère ***f*** **radiale** artery running along the radius

radiation ***f*** radiation

radiation ***f*** **ionisante** ionising radiation

radical ***m*** **libre** free (unchanging) radical (element/atom forming part of a chemical compound)

radiculaire ***adj*** relating to nerve root

conflit ***m*** **disco-radiculaire** spinal-cord nerve trapped by a slipped disc

radiesthésie ***f*** power of divination (using pendulum to locate body area affected)

radioactif -ive ***adj*** radioactive

radioactivité ***f*** radioactivity

radiographie ***f*** radiography; X-ray photography

passer ***v*** **une radiographie** to have an X-ray taken

radiographier to X-ray

se faire radiographier to have an X-ray taken

radiologie ***f*** radiology

radiologie ***f*** **interventionnelle** radiology used to visually follow path of small instruments in the body

radiologue/radiologiste ***m/f*** radiologist

radioscopie ***f*** radioscopy (X-ray examination of objects opaque to light)

radiothérapeute ***m/f*** radiotherapist

radiothérapie ***f*** radiotherapy (radiation treatment)

radius ***m*** radius (arm bone)

rage ***f*** rabies

vaccination ***f*** **antirabique** antirabies vaccination

rage ***f*** **de dents** toothache

raideur ***f*** stiffness

raideur ***f*** **de la nuque** stiff neck

raie ***f*** **des fesses** posterior rugae (cleft between the buttocks)

râle ***m*** rale (abnormal breathing sound)

ralentissement ***m*** slowing down (physical or organ functions)

ramollir ***v*** to soften

ramollissement ***m*** softening

ramollissement *m* cérébral stroke

rappel *m* booster (injection)

RAS (rien à signaler) nothing to report (on test results, etc.)

raser *v* to shave

rasoir *m* mécanique/de sûreté safety razor

rasoir *m* jetable disposable razor

rate *f* spleen

raviver *v* to reopen (cut, etc.)

Raynaud, syndrome *m* de Raynaud's syndrome (poor blood circulation)

rayon *m* de vision line of vision/of sight

rayon *m* ionisant ionising radiation

rayon *m* laser laser beam

rayonnant(e) *adj* spreading

rayonnement *m* infrarouge infrared radiation

rayonnement *m* ultraviolet ultraviolet radiation

rayons *mpl* gamma gamma rays; radiation

réaction *f* reaction

cuti-réaction *f* skin test

virage *m* d'une cuti-réaction positive reaction to a skin test (symptoms are present)

réaction *f* immunitaire body's natural defence reaction process

réadaptation *f* physique physical rehabilitation

réadapter *v* to readjust; to rehabilitate

réanimateur *m* resuscitator; respirator

réanimation *f* resuscitation

être *v* en réanimation to be in intensive care

service *m* de la réanimation intensive care unit

réanimer/ranimer *v* to resuscitate

recentrage *m* restoration (of dislocated bone/joint to its proper position)

réceptivité *f* susceptibility (to)

récessif -ive *adj* receding

receveur –euse *m/f* recipient

receveur –euse *m/f* universel(le) universal recipient

recherche *f* diagnostique diagnostic investigations (blood tests, observation)

rechute *f* relapse

avoir/faire *v* une rechute to have a relapse

rechuter *v* to relapse

récidivant(e) *adj* recurring (after complete recovery)

récidive *f* recurrence (of an illness)

récidiver *v* to recur

récidivité *f* recurring nature

recoudre *v* to stitch up again/to put stitches back in (wound); to stitch back up (after operation)

recouvrer *v* to recover; to regain (sight/view)

rectal(e) *adj* rectal

rectite *f* inflammation of the rectum

recto-colite *f* simultaneous inflammation of rectum and colon

recto-colite *f* hémorragique with bleeding from large intestine

rectoscope *m* rectoscope

rectoscopie *f* rectoscopy (internal examination of the rectum with rectoscope)

rectum *m* rectum

récupération *f* recovery; recuperation

récupérer *v* to recover; to recuperate

recurrent(e) *adj* recurrent

réductible *adj* fracture which can be reduced/set

réduction *f* setting/reduction of fracture

réduire *v* une facture to set/reduce a fracture

rééducation *f* rehabilitation; physiotherapy

centre *m* de rééducation rehabilitation centre

exercice *m* de rééducation physiotherapeutic exercise

faire *v* de la rééducation to undergo/have rehabilitation therapy

rééducation *f* de la parole speech therapy

rééduquer *v* to rehabilitate

réflexe *m* ostéo-tendineux automatic reflex (to doctor's reflex test)

réflexe ***m*** **palpébral** blinking reaction

réflexologie ***f*** reflexology (massage through reflex points)

reflux ***m*** reflux (return of liquid in the body)

reflux ***m*** **hépato-jugulaire** blood reflux from liver to jugular vein

reflux ***m*** **vésico-urétéral** urine reflux from bladder to kidneys

refroidissement ***m*** chill

attraper ***v*** **un refroidissement** to catch a chill

régénération ***f*** regeneration (tissues/cells)

régénérateur –trice ***adj*** regenerative

régime ***m*** diet

régime ***m*** **amaigrissant** slimming diet

suivre ***v*** **un régime** to be on a diet

région ***f*** area of the body

région ***f*** **lombaire** lumbar area

règles ***fpl*** period; menstruation

réglisse ***f*** liquorice

regonfler ***v*** to swell up again

régression ***f*** regression

régurgitation ***f*** regurgitation

réhydratation ***f*** moisturising (skin)

rehydrater ***v*** **(se)** to rehydrate (oneself); to moisturise (skin)

rein ***m*** kidney

rein ***m*** **artificiel** dialysis machine; kidney machine

avoir ***v*** **mal aux reins** to have backache

tour ***m*** **de reins** sprained/strained back

rejet ***m*** rejection (of graft/transplant)

relaxant ***m*** relaxant

relaxant(e) ***adj*** relaxing

relaxation ***f*** relaxation

remaniement ***m*** modification (of organ, following illness)

remboursement ***m*** refund; reimbursement

remède ***m*** remedy; medicine; ointment

remède ***m*** **hémorroïdaire** ointment for haemorrhoids

rémission ***f*** remission; abatement

rémittent(e) ***adj*** remittent (abates from time to time)

remnographie ***f*** **(**using **résonance** ***f*** **magnétique**

nucléaire) 3D electro-magnetic medical imagery exam

remontant ***m*** tonic (booster); antidepressant

remplaçant(e) ***m/f*** locum; replacement

rénal(e) ***adj*** renal

défaillance ***f*****/insuffisance** ***f*** **rénale** renal/kidney failure

insuffisance ***f*** **rénale aiguë** acute renal/kidney failure

repérage ***f*** location (of lesion)

réplétion ***f*** repletion (e.g. of stomach)

(se) reposer ***v*** to rest

résection ***f*** resection (surgical removal of section/part of organ)

résidence ***f*** **médicalisée** nursing home

résorber ***v*** to reabsorb (liquid/surgical thread)

résoudre ***v*** to resolve (remove tumour etc.)

respirateur ***m*** **artificel** respirator; ventilator

respiration ***f*** breathing; respiration

respiration ***f*** **artificielle** artificial respiration

respiration ***f*** **assistée** assisted ventilation

respiration ***f*** **bruyante/sifflante** wheezing

respiratoire ***adj*** respiratory

appareil ***m*** **respiratoire** respiratory tract

arrêt ***m*** **respiratoire** respiratory failure

kinésithérapie ***f*** **respiratoire** breathing exercises

système ***m*** **respiratoire** respiratory system

respirer to breathe

respirer ***v*** **avec difficulté** to have difficulty breathing

respirez ***imp*** breathe in

rester ***v*** to stay; to remain

rester ***v*** **éveillé** to keep/stay awake

rester ***v*** **sans bouger/sans rien dire** to stay/remain motionless/silent

rester ***v*** **dans la gorge** to stick in the throat

rester ***v*** **handicapé(e) à vie** to be handicapped for life

y rester ***v*** **(colloquial)** to die

(se) rétablir ***v*** to recuperate
rétention ***f*** retention
rétine ***f*** retina
rétinite ***f*** retinitis (retina inflammation)
rétinite ***f*** **pigmentaire** pigmentary retinitis (congenital condition leading to blindness)
rétinopathie ***f*** retinal diseases (other than retinitis)
rétrécissement ***m*** contraction (muscle, retina); shrinking; stricture (narrowing of canal/ duct in body)
rétrécissement ***m*** **aortique (RA)** narrowing of aortic (heart) valve
rétrécissement ***m*** **mitral (RM)** narrowing of mitral (heart) valve
rétroversé(e) ***adj*** retroverted (e.g. of the womb)
rétrovirus ***m*** retrovirus (including the Aids virus)
rêve ***m*** dream
révulsif -ive ***adj*** revulsive
révulsion ***f*** revulsion (counterirritation treatment)
rhésus ***m*** **positif/négatif** rhesus (Rh) positive/negative (blood group)
facteur rhésus ***m*** rhesus or Rh factor
rhinite ***f*** rhinitis (inflammation of nose)
rhinopharyngite ***f*** rhinopharyngitis (sore nose and throat)
rhumatismal ***adj*** rheumatic
rhumatisme ***m*** rheumatism
rhumatisme ***m*** **articulaire** articular rheumatism (in the joints)
rhumatisme ***m*** **chronique polyarticulaire** rheumatoid arthritis
rhumatisme ***m*** **déformant** polyarthritis
rhumatoïde ***adj*** rheumatoid
rhumatologie ***f*** rheumatology
rhumatologiste ***m/f*** rheumatologist
rhume ***m*** cold
rhume ***m*** **chronique** catarrh
rhume ***m*** **de cerveau** head cold
rhume ***m*** **des foins** ***m*** hay fever
rhume ***m*** **de hanche** temporary swelling of hip area and

feverous condition affecting children

riboflavine ***f*** riboflavin (vitamin B)

ride ***f*** wrinkle

rigidité ***f*** **cadavérique** rigor mortis

romarin ***m*** rosemary (tonic)

ronflement ***m*** snoring

ronfler to snore

rosacée ***f*** rosacea (red acne)

roséole ***f*** roseola (rosy rash)

Risser, score/test de ***m*** Risser's growth chart (from birth to maturity)

RLS (abbreviation of **restless legs syndrome** ***m*****)** restless legs syndrome

RM (abbreviation of **rétrécissement mitral** ***m*****)** see above

rotateur ***m*** rotator (muscle)

coiffe ***f*** **des rotateurs** ***mpl*** shoulder muscle tendons

rotateur ***adj*** rotative (muscle)

rotule ***f*** patella; kneecap

rougeole ***f*** measles

rougeur ***m*** rash; redness; red blotch/patch

ruban ***m*** **de tissu adhésif** adhesive tape

rubéole ***f*** German measles

rupture ***f*** rupture

rupture ***f*** **tendineuse** rupture or tearing of a tendon

rythme ***m*** **du coeur** heart rate

rythme ***m*** **cardiaque** rate of heartbeat

saccharine ***f*** saccharin

saccharose ***m*** saccharose; sucrose

sacrum ***m*** sacrum (bone between the two hip bones)

sage-femme ***f*** midwife

saignée ***f*** bleeding; blood letting

saignement ***m*** bleeding

saignement ***m*** **de nez** nose bleed

temps ***m*** **de saignement** bleeding time before coagulation

saigner to bleed

saillant(e) ***adj*** bulging (when concerning eyes); prominent; protruding

salive ***f*** saliva

salle ***f*** **d'examen** examination room

salle ***f*** **d'hôpital** hospital ward

salle ***f*** **d'opération** operating theatre

salmonelle ***f*** salmonella

salmonellose ***f*** salmonella food poisoning

salpingectomie ***f*** salpingectomy (surgical removal of Fallopian tubes)

salpingite ***f*** salpingitis (inflammation of Fallopian tube or the Eustachian [ear] tube)

sanatorium ***m*** sanatorium

sang ***m*** blood

dérivés ***mpl*****/produits** ***mpl*** **du sang/produits** ***mpl*** **sanguins** blood derivatives/products (platelets, red corpuscles, etc.)

sang ***m*** **contaminé** contaminated blood

sanitaires ***mpl*** bathrooms; washrooms

sanitaire ***adj*** health; sanitary

santé ***f*** health

santé ***f*** **mentale** mental health

en bonne/mauvaise santé ***f*** in good/bad health

sapeur-pompier ***m*** fireman

saphène ***f*** saphena; (saphenous vein)

sarcoïdose ***f*** sarcodosis (disease resembling TB)

sarcome ***m*** sarcoma (malignant tumour)

saturnisme ***m*** saturnism (lead poisoning)

saturométrie ***f*** oxygen or carbon dioxide level measurement in the blood

sauge ***f*** salvia (healing plant)

sauna ***m*** sauna

sauvetage ***m*** rescue

cours ***m*** **de sauvetage** life-saving lessons

savon ***m*** soap

savon ***m*** **de Marseille** household soap

savon ***m*** **100 pour cent végétal** 100 per cent vegetable content soap

savon ***m*** **dermatologique** dermatological soap

savon ***m*** **de toilette** toilet soap

savon ***m*** **pour bébé** baby soap

scabieux -euse ***adj*** scabby; affected with mange

scalpel ***m*** scalpel

scanner ***m*****/scanneur** ***m*** scanner

scanographe ***m*** scanner **(exclusively medical term)**

passer *v* un scanner/ scanographe to have a scan

scapulaire *m* shoulder blade; scapula

scapulaire *adj* scapular

ceinture *f* scapulaire pectoral girdle

scarificateur *m* scarificator (scalpel for small incisions)

scarifier *v* to scarify

scarlatine *f* scarlet fever

Scheuermann, maladie de *f* Scheuermann's disease (deformation of spinal column)

schistosomiase *f* bilharzia ('worms')

schizophrène *adj* schizophrenic

schizophrénie *f* schizophrenia

sciatique *f* sciatica

sciatique *adj* sciatic

scintigraphie *f* scintigraphy (2D medical imagery using gamma rays)

scissure *f* interhémisphérique longitudinal fissure of the brain

sclérodermie *f* scleroderma (chronic skin and tissue hardening)

sclérose *f* sclerosis

sclérose *f* artérielle hardening of the arteries; arteriosclerosis

sclérose *f* en plaques multiple sclerosis

sclérose *f* multiple multiple sclerosis

se scléroser *v* to become sclerotic

sclérotique *adj* sclerotic

sclérotique *f* sclera (white of the eye)

scoliose *f* scoliosis (curvature of the spine)

scoliose *f* dextroconvexe spine curvature to the right

scoliose *f* sinistroconvexe spine curvature to the left

scorbut *m* scurvy

scorbutique *adj* scorbutic (affected with scurvy)

scotch-test *m* scotch test (biological test in anal area)

scrofule *f* scrofula (condition with glandular swellings)

scrotal(e) *adj* scrotal

scrotum *m* scrotum

séance *f* session (exercise, treatment)

sébacé(e) *adj* sebaceous (fatty: of skin)

glande *f* sébacée sebaceous gland
séborrhée *f* seborrhoea (excessive discharge of sebum)
sécable *adj* divisible or scored (pill, tablet)
secondaire *adj* concerning secondary illness caused by a previous one; side-effects of medicine
sébum *m* sebum (sebaceous glands secretion)
sécheresse *f* cutanée dryness of the skin
sécheresse *f* oculaire dryness of the eyes
secret *m* médical medical confidentiality
sécrétion *f* secretion
secteur *m* part of an organ
sédatif *m* sedative
sédatif -ive *adj* sedative
sédation *f* sedation
sédentaire *adj* sedentary
sédiment *m* sediment
sédimentation *f* sedimentation
sein *m* breast
cancer du sein *m* breast cancer
sel de Glauber *m* Glauber's salt (sodium sulphate)
selles *fpl* stools; motions
aller *v* à la selle to have/pass a motion
semence *f* semence; sperm
séminal *adj* seminal (of/concerning semen)
sénile *adj* senile
sénilité *f* senility
sénologie *f* study of the breast
sénologue *m* breast specialist
sens *m* sense
sensation *f* sensation
sensibilisation *f* sensitisation
sensibilisé(e) *adj* sensitised
sensibilité *f* sensitivity
sensitif -ive *adj* sensitive
sentir *v* to feel; to smell
ne pas se sentir *v* bien to not feel well
septal(e) *adj* of septum
septum *m* septum (body partition)
septicémie *f* septacemia (septic poisoning)
septicité *f*; état *m* septique septicity
septique *adj* septic (fever/bacteria)
séquelle *f* after-effect

séquelle ***f*** **indemnisable** consequences which can be sued for

séquestre ***m*** bone fragment (following necrosis)

sérénité ***f*** serenity

séreuse ***f*** membrane (covering certain organs)

séreux -euse ***adj*** serous (containing serum)

seringue ***f*** syringe

seringue ***f*** **pour injections** hypodermic syringe

sérique ***adj*** relating to blood serum

sérologie ***f*** serology; tests for blood disease symptoms

séronégatif -ive ***adj*** seronegative (negative blood test result)

séropositif -ive ***adj*** seropositive (positive blood test result)

sérotonine ***f*** serotonin (compound in blood platelets and serum acting as neurotransmitter); drug group aiding sleep and depressive disorders

sérum ***m*** serum

sérum ***m*** **antidiphthérique** antidiphtheria serum

sérum ***m*** **antitétanique** antitetanus serum

sérum ***m*** **antivenimeux** snakebite serum

sérum ***m*** **artificiel/ physiologique** physiological serum/salt solution

sérum ***m*** **sanguin** blood serum

service ***m*** (hospital) ward; department

service ***m*** **ambulancier** ambulance service

service ***m*** **d'accouchement** maternity department; obstetric department

service ***m*** **d'obstétrique** obstetric department

service ***m*** **d'oto-rhino-laryngologie** ear, nose and throat department

service ***m*** **de cancer** cancer ward

service ***m*** **de gastro-entérologie** gastro-enterology department

service ***m*** **d'imagerie médicale** medical imagery department

service *m* de maternité maternity ward
service *m* de pédiatrie paediatrics ward
service *m* gériatrique geriatric ward
service *m* radiologique X-ray department
serviette *f* hygiénique sanitary towel
séton *m* à mèche seton; surgical cotton for wound drainage
seuil *m* auditif auditory threshold
seuil auditif *m* de la douleur: 120 dB auditory pain threshold: 120 decibels (DB)
sevrage *m* weaning
sevrage *m* pharmacologique drug substitute (for drug addicts)
symptômes *mpl* de sevrage withdrawal symptoms
sexe *m* sex; genitals
sexologue *m/f* sex therapist
sexualité *f* sexuality
sexué(e) *adj* possessing a sex; sexual
sexuel(le) *adj* sexual
shampooing *m*/shampoing *m* shampoo
shampooing *m*/shampoing *m* pour bébé baby shampoo
shampooing *m*/shampoing *m* traitant fortifiant fortifying treatment shampoo
shunt *m* shunt (surgical creation of alternative passage for blood circulation)
shunt *m* artério-veineux surgical shunt (surgically created passage for blood flow directly from artery to vein)
sibilant(e) *adj* sibilant (hissing/whistling sound)
SIDA *m* (syndrome immunodéficitaire acquis) AIDS (acquired immune deficiency syndrome)
siège *m* complet complete/full breech birth presentation
siège *m* décomplété frank (unmistakeable) breech birth presentation
siège *m* de bain waterproof chair for the bath
siège *m* réhausseur booster seat (for toilet seats)

sifflement ***m*** whistling/hissing (ears)

sigmoïde ***m*** **(**abbrev. of **colon** ***m*** **sigmoïde)** sigmoid colon (penultimate part of large intestine)

sigmoïde ***adj*** of/concerning sigmoid colon

sigmoïdectomie ***f*** sigmoidectomy (removal of sigmoid colon)

signe ***m*** **clinique** clinical sign

signe ***m*** **de Lachman** Lachman's sign (tibia pulls forward or backward more than normal)

significatif -ive ***adj*** significant

silicone ***f*** silicon

silicose ***f*** silicosis (miners' lung disease)

sinus ***m*** sinus

sinus ***m*** **carotidien** carotid sinusitis (swelling of either of two main arteries to the neck and head)

sillon ***m*** fissure

sinusite ***f*** sinusitis

siphon ***m*** siphon

sirop ***m*** **antitussif** cough mixture/syrup

sirop ***m*** **pour la toux** cough syrup/mixture

soif ***f*** thirst

soigner to treat illness/patient

(se) soigner to take medicine

soins ***mpl*** treatment; care; after-care

soins ***mpl*** **corporels** body care

soins ***mpl*** **dentaires** dental care

soins ***mpl*** **des cheveux** hair care

soins ***mpl*** **de pédicure/du pied** chiropody

soins ***mpl*** **des ongles** nail care

soins ***mpl*** **intensifs** intensive care

soins ***mpl*** **médicaux** health/medical care

soins ***mpl*** **nettoyants** cleansing treatments

soins ***mpl*** **palliatifs** palliative/pain alleviating care

solaire ***adj*** (of) sun

crème ***f*** **solaire** suntan cream

émulsion ***f*** **solaire** suntan emulsion

huile ***f*** **solaire** suntan oil

lotion ***f*** **solaire** suntan lotion

spray ***m*** **solaire** suntan spray

soluté ***m*** solution

solution ***f*** solution

solution ***f*** **de continuité** surgical incision; accidental cut or rupture
solution ***f*** **oculaire** eye solution
solution ***f*** **de rinçage** rinsing solution
solution ***f*** **de stérilisation** sterilising solution
en solution in solution form
sommeil ***m*** sleep
somnambule ***m/f*** sleepwalker
somnambulisme ***m*** sleepwalking
somatique ***adj*** somatic
maladie ***f*** **somatique** illness with physical cause
somnifère ***m*** sleeping pill
somnolence ***f*** drowsiness
somnoler ***v*** to doze
son nocif ***m*** harmful noise
sondage ***m*** probe; catheterisation
sonde ***f*** probe
sonde ***f*** **d'alimentation** feeding tube
sonde ***f*** **creuse/à canal central** catheter
sonde ***f*** **gastrique** stomach tube
sonde ***f*** **urétrale** urethral tube
sonder ***v*** to probe (wound); to catheterise (bladder)
sophrologie ***f*** relaxation therapy
soporifique ***adj*** soporific
sortie ***f*** patient discharge (release from hospital)
souffle ***m*** **cardiaque** cardiac murmur
souffle ***m*** **au cœur** heart murmur
souffrant(e) ***adj*** unwell
souffrir to suffer
soulager to ease; to relieve
sourcil ***m*** eyebrow
sourd(e) ***adj*** deaf
sous-alimentation ***f*** malnutrition
sous-crépitant ***adj*** spluttering (sound from lungs)
sparadrap ***m*** medical adhesive tape; plaster
sparadrap ***m*** **microporeux** microporous adhesive tape
spasme ***m*** spasm
spasme ***m*** **clonique** involuntary intense spasms
spasmophilie ***f*** involuntary facial and arm spasms
spatule ***f*** spatula
spécialiste ***m/f*** specialist

spécifique ***adj*** characteristically specific (symptom)

speculum ***m*** speculum (surgical inspection instrument)

sperme ***m*** semen; sperm

spermicide ***m*** spermicide

spermicide ***adj*** spermicidal

spermogramme ***m*** sperm count and analysis

sphincter ***m*** sphincter

sphincter ***m*** **anal** anal sphincter

sphygmomanomètre ***m*** sphygmomanometer (instrument that measures blood pressure)

sphygmomanomètre ***m*** **électronique de poignet** wrist sphygmomanometer

spina-bifida ***m*** spina bifida

spina-bifida ***m*** **occulta** mild spina bifida

spirométrie ***f*** measurement of lungs air capacity (using a spirometer)

spironolactone ***m*** diuretic medicine/drug

splénectomie ***f*** splenectomy (surgical removal of the spleen)

splénomégalie ***f*** oversized spleen

spondylarthrite ***f*** **ankylosante** ankylosing spondylitis (inflammation and stiffening of the vertebrae)

spondylite ***f*** spondylitis (inflammation of a vertebra)

spondylopathie ***f*** spondylopathy (spinal disease)

spore ***f*** spore (reproductive cell)

spray ***m*** spray (aerosol/vaporiser)

sprue ***f*** sprue (tropical disease)

sputum ***m*** spit

squame ***f*** scale (skin); squama

squameux -euse ***adj*** scaly; squamous

dermatose ***f*** **squameuse** (scaly) skin disease

squelette ***f*** skeleton

SRAS (syndrome ***m*** **respiratoire aigu sévère)** SARS (severe acute respiratory syndrome)

stade ***m*** stage (of illness)

stage ***m*** course (of treatment)

staphylococcie ***f*** staphylococcia

staphylocoque ***m*** staphylococcus (bacterium, sometimes causing pus formation)

staphylococque *m* doré staphyloccus aureus (grape-like formation)
stase *f* stasis (stoppage/slowing down of circulation of any of the body fluids)
stase *f* stercorale constipation
statines *fpl* medicines/drugs for cholesterol
station *f* thermale spa
staturo-pondéral(e) *adj* concerning both height and weight
développement *m* staturo-pondéral child's height-weight development (chart)
stéatopygie *f* steatopygy (fattiness in female buttocks)
sténose *f* stenosis (abnormal narrowing of passage in body)
stent *m* stent (metal tube used to widen arteries)
steppage *m* shuffling gait
stepper *m* stepping exercise machine
stérile *adj* sterile
stérilet *m* intra-uterine coil
stérilisateur *m* steriliser
stérilisation *f* sterilisation
stériliser *v* to sterilise
stérilité *f* sterility
sternum *m* sternum
stéroïde *m* steroid
stéroïde *m* hormonal steroidal hormone
stéthoscope *m* stethoscope
stick *m* stick (cosmetics, cream, etc.)
stigmate *m* stigma; mark; scar
stimulateur *m* cardiaque; stimulateur artificiel pacemaker
stomacal *adj* of/concerning the stomach
stomatite *f* stomatis (inflammation of the mouth)
stomatologie *f* stomatology (study of mouth and teeth or their diseases)
stomatologue *m/f* stomatologist
stomie *f* stomach bag operation
strabisme *m* strabismus (one or both eyes out of normal position)
strapping *m* support bandage
streptocoque *m* streptococcus (bacterium)
streptocoque *m* bêta-hémolytique streptococcus

(causing scarlet fever, acute articular rheumatism)
streptomycine ***f*** streptomycin (antibiotic)
stress ***m*** stress
stressant(e) ***adj*** stressful
stresser to stress; to put under stress
stretching ***m*** stretching exercises
stripping ***m*****/éveinage** ***m*** varicose vein removal
stromal(e) (***pl*** **-aux)** ***adj*** relating to alimentary canal
stupéfiant ***m*** drug; narcotic
stupéfiant(e) ***adj*** stupefying
stupéfier to stupefy
stupeur ***f*** stupor
stylet ***m*** stylet; stilette (small probe)
subcophose ***f*** partial deafness
substitutif ***m*** **hormonal** hormone substitute (post-menopause)
succion ***f*** suction; sucking
sucette ***f*** baby's dummy; comforter
sucre ***m*** **dans le sang** blood sugar level
sucres ***mpl*** **lents** complex sugars
sudamina ***m*****; boutons** ***m*** **de chaleur** sudamina; heat spots
sudation ***f*** perspiration; sweat
sueur ***f*** perspiration; sweat
suffocation ***f*** choking; suffocation
avoir ***v*** **des suffocations** to have choking fits
sulfamide ***m*** sulphonamide (sulphonic acid derivative)
supplémenter ***v*** **une alimentation** to balance an unbalanced diet
suppositoire ***m*** suppository
suppuration ***f*** suppuration (formation of pus)
suppurer ***v*** to suppurate
sural(e) ***adj*** relating to calf muscle
suralimentation ***f*** feeding up (therapy); overeating
suralimenter ***v*** to feed up
(se) suralimenter ***v*** to overeat
surcharge ***f*** **pondérale** excess weight (too much for good health)
surdi-mutité ***f*** deaf-and-dumbness
surdité ***f*** deafness
surdosage ***m*** overdose

surdose *f* overdose
surgétique *f* surgetics (computer-aided surgery)
surinfection *f* secondary infection
surmenage *m* **intellectuel** mental fatigue
surmenage *m* **physique** overexertion
surmonter to overcome (illness)
surpoids *m* overweight; surplus weight
sursiège *m*; **soutien dos** ergonomic seat cover for back support
surveillance *f* **électronique** electronic monitoring
surveillance *f* **médicale** medical supervision
surveillant(e) *m/f* head/chief nurse; charge nurse
surveillante *f* **générale** matron
sustenter *v* to sustain (with food)
suture *f* suture; seam-like junction of two bones
suturer *v* to suture; to stitch up
sycosis *f* sycosis (facial disease in bearded area)
symptôme *m* symptom (change felt by patient)
symptôme(s) *m* **actif(s)** *adj* active, manifest sign(s) of an illness
synapse *f* synapse (neurotransmission gap between two nerve cells)
syncope *f* blackout; fainting fit
tomber *v* **en syncope** to blackout; to faint
syndrome *m* syndrome
syndrome *m* **d'Asperger** Asperger's syndrome (atypical personality development)
syndrome *m* **de Down** Down's syndrome
syndrome *m* **du choc toxique (SCT)** Toxic Shock Syndrome (TSS)
syndrome *m* **immunodéficitaire acquis (SIDA)** acquired immunodeficiency syndrom (AIDS)
syndrome *m* **des jambes sans repos (SJSR)** restless legs syndrome (RLS)
syndrome *m* **obstructif pulmonaire** syndrome due to

difficult passage of air through the lungs

syndrome *m* obstructif rénal urine passage difficulty from kidneys to bladder

syndrome *m* occlusif signs of intestinal blockage

syndrome *m* prémenstruel (PMS) premenstrual sydrome (PMS)

syndrome *m* respiratoire aigu sévère (SRAS) severe acute respiratory syndrome (SARS)

syndrome de Raynaud Raynaud's syndrome (poor blood circulation)

synergie *f* synergy

synergiste *m* synergist (medicine or organ working with another)

synergiste *adj* synergistic

synoviale *f* synovial membrane (around joints)

synovite *f* synovitis (inflammation of the synovial membrane)

syphilis *f* syphilis

système *m* system

système *m* cardio-vasculaire cardio-vascular system

système *m* digestif digestive system

système *m* endocrinien endocrine system (glands)

système *m* immunitaire immune system

système *m* lymphatique lymphatic system

système *m* nerveux autonome autonomic nervous system

système *m* nerveux central central nervous system (brain, spinal cord)

système *m* nerveux périphérique peripheral nervous system

système *m* parasympathique parasympathetic nervous system (from brain to lower spinal cord)

système *m* pileux très développé a lot of body hair

système *m* respiratoire respiratory system

systémique *adj* systemic (concerning the whole body)

maladie *f* systémique systemic illness (illness which spreads throughout the body, but with little known origin)

systole *f* systole (intervals between heart contractions when blood is pumped into arteries)
diastole *f* diastole (intervals between heart contractions when the chambers fill with blood)

tabagique ***adj*** concerning tobacco use
intoxication *f* **tabagique** tobacco poisoning
dépendance *f* **tabagique** smoking addiction
tabagique ***f/m*** chain smoker
tabagisme ***m*** smoking addiction; nicotine addiction
tabagisme ***m*** **passif** passive smoking (inhalation of other people's cigarette smoke)
tableau ***m*** **d'acuité visuelle** sight testing chart
tableau ***m*** **clinique** clinical picture (observations)
tache *f* **aveugle** blind spot
tache *f* **café-au-lait** brown mark on skin
tache *f* **de naissance** birthmark
tache *f* **de son** strawberry mark
tache *f* **polychrome** ***adj*** multi-coloured spot (may be beginning of a cancer)
taches ***fpl*** **rouges** red spots
tachyarythmie *f* tachyarrythmia (irregular heartbeat with fast bursts)
tachycardie *f* tachycardia (abnormally fast heart rate)
tachycardie *f* **jonctionnelle** heart rate illness due to disorder in the heart's nerve centre
Tai-chi-chuan; Tai-ji-quan ***m*** t'ai chi
taie *f* leucoma (white opacity in the cornea)
taille *f* waist/waistline; waist size (clothes)
talc ***m*** talcum powder
talon ***m*** heel
tapis ***m*** **roulant** treadmill exerciser
tampon ***m*** swab; pad buffer
tampon ***m*** **hygiénique** tampon
tamponnement ***m*** tamponade; tamponage (compression of the heart disorder)
tapotement ***m*** tapotement; percussion massage

tapoter ***v*** to tap

tarse ***m*** tarsus (the group of ankle and upper foot bones)
  os ***m*** **du tarse** tarsal bone

tartre ***m*** tartar

tassement ***m*** **de la colonne vertébrale** compression of the spinal column

tatouage ***m*** tattoo; tattooing

taux ***m*** level

taux ***m*** **de cholestérol** cholesterol level

taux ***m*** **d'alcoolémie** amount of alcohol in the blood

TC (abbreviation of **traumatisme crânien)** see below

TDM (abbreviation of **tonsodensiométrie)** see below

tégument ***m*** tegument (skin, body hair)

teigne ***f*** tinea; ringworm

teinture ***f*** **d'arnica/d'iodine** arnica/iodine tincture

téléradiographie ***f*** teleradiography (X-rays from a certain distance for increased precision)

téléradiothérapie ***f*** teleradiotherapy

temporal ***m*** temporal (temple) bone

température ***f*** temperature
  avoir/faire ***v*** **de la température** to have a temperature
  prendre ***v*** **la température** to take (someone's) temperature

temps ***m*** **de coagulation** coagulation time

temps ***m*** **de latence** latent/incubation period

temps de saignement bleeding time

tendon ***m*** tendon; sinew

tendon ***m*** **d'Achille** Achille's tendon

tendinite ***f*** tendinitis (inflammation of the tendon); enthésiopathie *f*

teneur ***m*** **du sang en alcool éthylique** alcohol content in blood

tenir ***v*** to keep; to stock

tenir ***v*** **hors de la portée et de la vue des enfants** keep out of children's reach and view

ténia ***m*****/taenia** ***m*** tapeworm; taenia

tensiomètre ***m*** sphygmomanometer (instrument that measures blood pressure)

tensiomètre ***m*** **électronique de poignet** electronic, wrist sphygmomanometer

tension ***f*** **artérielle** blood pressure

tension ***f*** **artérielle diastolique/systolique** diastolic/systolic blood pressure

tension ***f*** **intraoculaire/oculaire** intraocular blood pressure

tension ***f*** **montée/baissée** raised/lowered blood pressure

prendre ***v*** **la tension** to take blood pressure

souffrir ***v*** **d'hypertension** to suffer from high blood pressure

trop de tension ***f*** hypertension

vérifier ***v*** **la tension** to check blood pressure

hypertension/hypotension ***f*** high/low blood pressure

tente ***f*** tent-like membrane adjacent to the cerebellum

tente ***f*** **à oxygène** oxygen tent

tépographie ***f*** 3D medical imagery indicating how organs are functioning

tératogène ***adj*** teratogenic (of illnesses/medicines suffered/taken in early pregnancy which can produce malformation in babies)

terme ***m*** term

accouchement ***m*** **à terme** full-term childbirth

accoucher ***v*** **avant terme** to give birth prematurely

terrain ***m*** body susceptible to illnesses

tertiaire ***adj*** tertiary

test ***m*** **d'acuité visuelle** eyesight test

test ***m*** **d'allergie** allergy test

test ***m*** **de grossesse** pregnancy test

test ***m*** **psychologique** psychological test

testicule ***m*** testicule

testostérone ***f*** testosterone (male hormone)

tétanie ***f*** tetany (muscle spasm)

tétanos ***m*** tetanus

tête ***f*** head

tête ***f*** **de l'humérus** shoulder end of the humerus bone

tétine ***f*** teat (baby's bottle); dummy

donner ***v*** **à téter à un bébé** to breast-feed a baby

tétracycline ***f*** tetracyline (type of antibiotic)

tétralogie ***f*** **de Fallot** Fallot's congenital heart-valve malformation

tétraplégique ***m/f and adj*** quadriplegic; tetraplegic (person with total limb paralysis)

thalamus ***m*** thalamus (darker tissues of forebrain)

thalassothérapie ***f*** thalassotherapy; sea-water therapy

thalassémie ***f*** thalassemia (illness at birth due to lack of red corpuscles)

théâtre ***m*** **d'opérations** operating theatre

théophylline ***f*** tea alkaloid with diuretic and dilation (of bronchial tubes) properties

thérapeutique ***f*** therapeutics; treatment

thérapeutique ***adj*** therapeutic

substance ***f*** **thérapeutique** medicine

thérapeutiques ***fpl*** **diverses** therapeutics/treatments (classed as alternative/non-conventional medicine)

thérapie ***f*** therapy

thérapie ***f*** **de groupe** group therapy

thérapie ***f*** **génique** gene therapy

thérapie ***f*** **institutionnelle** institutional therapy (treatment over a period of time in a psychiatric home)

suivre ***v*** **une thérapie** to follow/take course of treatment

thermalisme ***m*** water cures

thermoformage ***m*** thermal compression moulding (chiropodist's false soles, etc.)

thermomètre ***m*** thermometer

thermomètre ***m*** **à infrarouges** infrared thermometer

thermomètre ***m*** **à maxima et minima** maximum and minimum thermometer

thermomètre *m* à mercure/ alcool mercury/alcohol thermometer

thermomètre *m* électronique electronic thermometer

thermomètre *m* médical clinical thermometer

thermothérapie *f* thermotherapy (heat treatment)

thorax *m* thorax

thoractomie *f* operation to open stomach

thrombine *f* thrombin (causes blood clotting)

thrombose *f* thrombosis

thrombose *f* coronarienne coronary thrombosis

thymique *adj* thymic (of/ concerning the thymus)

thymus *m* thymus (neck gland)

thyroïde *f* thyroid

thyroïde *adj* thyroid

tibia *m* tibia (shin bone)

tic *m* tic

timbre *m* transdermique medicated skin plaster/patch (such as nicotine patch)

tirer *v* la langue to put the tongue out

tiroir *m* du genou anterior drawer sign of knee (tibia pulls forward or backward more than normal)

tissu *m* tissue

tissu *m* adipeux fatty tissue

tissu *m* cicatriciel scar tissue

tissu *m* conjonctif connective tissue

tissu *m* épithélial epithelial tissue (body and digestive tract tissue)

tissu *m* musculaire muscular tissue

tissu *m* osseux bone tissue

titane *m* titanium (used in prostheses)

toise *f* height gauge/chart

tolérance *f* tolerance (to treatment or to receptivity of graft)

tolérer *v* to tolerate

tomber *v* to fall

tomber *v* dans le coma to fall into a coma

tomber *v* dans les pommes (informal) to faint/pass out

tomographie *f* tomography (3D medical imagery/scanning)

tomodensitométrie *f* scanning (of body)

tonicité *f* (body) tone; tonicity; muscle elasticity

tonique *m* tonic

tonique *adj* tonic

tonsille *f* tonsil

tonsillite *f*; **amygdalite** *f* tonsillitis

tonsillectomie *f* tonsillectomy (surgical removal of tonsils)

topique *m* **and** *adj* local/topical (medicine/pain/anaesthetic)

torsion *f* torsion

torticolis *m* torticollis; wryneck; stiff neck

toucher *m* **rectal/vaginal** rectal/vaginal finger probe

tourista *f* tourist's diarrhoea

tourniquet *m* tourniquet

tousser to cough

toux *f* cough; coughing

toux *f* **du fumeur** smoker's cough

toux *f* **grasse** loose cough

toux *f* **nerveuse** nervous cough

toux *f* **sèche** dry cough

toxémie *f* toxaemia; blood poisoning; increased blood pressure in pregnancy

toxicologie *f* toxicology

toxicologue *m/f* toxicologist (poison specialist)

toxicomane *m/f* drug addict

toxicomane *adj* drug-addicted

toxicomanie *f* drug addiction

toxine *f* toxin (produced by living organism)

toxique *adj* toxic

toxoplasmose *f* toxiplasmosis (parasitical infection)

trac *m* patient's pre-operation or pre-examination nerves

trace *f* scar; mark; very small amount (biology)

trachéal(e) *adj* tracheal (of/concerning the windpipe)

trachée-artère *f*; **trachée** *f* windpipe

trachéite *f* windpipe inflammation

trachéotomie *f*; **intubation** *f* **trachéale** tracheotomy

trachome *m* trachoma (eye infection)

tractus *m* tract (area of an organ or body system)

traitement *m* treatment

traitement *m* **adjuvant** secondary treatment

traitement *m* ambulatoire outpatient treatment

traitement *m* dentaire dental treatment

traitement *m* d'entretien sustaining treatment (to consolidate the cure)

traitement *m* palliatif palliative/pain-relieving treatment (for the terminally ill)

traiter *v* to treat

tranchées *fpl* colic; gripes

tranchées *fpl* utérines postnatal pain

tranquille *adj* calm

tranquillisant *m* tranquilliser

tranquillisant(e) *m/f and adj* soothing; tranquillising

transfuser *v* to transfuse

transfusion *f* sanguine blood transfusion

transgénique *adj* transgenic (such as foodstuff with genetically modified animal or vegetable content)

transit *m* intestinal digestion; intestinal transition

transmettre *v* to pass on/ transmit (illness)

transpiration *f* perspiration; sweat

transplantation *f* transplantation; transport

transplantation *f* cardiaque/ du rein heart/kidney transplant

transplanter *v* to transplant

transposition *f* congenital malformation of an organ; operation to displace the extremity of a tendon, artery, etc.

trauma *m* trauma

traumatique *adj* traumatic

traumatisme *m* traumatism

traumatisme crânien *m* cranial trauma

travail *m* childbirth; labour

traversin *m* bolster (for neck, head, back support)

tremblement *m* trembling; shaking

trembler *v* to tremble; to shake; to shiver

trémor *m* trembling

trémulation *f* tremor

trépan *m* surgical bore for trepanation

trépanation *f* trepanation (surgical opening of bone, esp. skull)

trépied *m* **méningitique** the three symptoms of meningitis

triceps *m* triceps

tricostéril *m* sterile compress

trisomie 21 *f* trisomy 21; Down's syndrome

trisomique *f* person with Down's syndrome

triglycéride *m* trigylceride (fat compounds in the blood)

trithérapie *f* three complementary medicines as treatment

trompe de Fallope *f* Fallopian tube

tronc *m* trunk

trouble *m* disorder

trouble du caractère *m* personality disorder

trouble *m* **fonctionnel** functional disorder

trouble *m* **du langage** speech difficulty

trouble *m* **obsessionnel compulsif** obsessive compulsive disorder

trouble *m* **trophique** organ/tissue malfunction through oxygen deficiency and malnourishment

trouble *m* **de la vision** eyesight trouble

trouble *m* **musculosquelettique** repetitive strain injury

trousse *f* **de premier secours** first-aid kit

trousse *f* **à pharmacie** first-aid kit

trousse *f* **de premier soins** first-aid kit

trousse *f* **d'urgence** first-aid box

tubage *m* intubation; surgical introduction of a cannula

tubaire *adj* tubal (relating to Fallopian tube)

tube *m* **digestif** alimentary canal

tubercule *m* tubercle (small rounded protuberance or swelling)

tuberculeux -euse *adj* tuberculous; tubercular

tuberculose *f* tuberculosis

tuméfaction *f* tumefaction; swelling/puffing up

tumeur ***f*** tumor
tympan ***m*** eardrum
typhoïde ***f*****; fièvre** ***f*** **typhoïde** typhoid; typhoid fever
typhus ***m*** typhus

ulcération ***f*** ulceration
ulcère ***m*** ulcer
ulcère ***m*** **de l'estomac** peptic ulcer; gastric ulcer
ulcère ***m*** **du duodénum** duodenal ulcer
ulcère ***m*** **variqueux** varicose ulcer
ulcérer ***v*** to ulcerate
ulcéreux -euse ***adj*** festering (wound); ulcerated
ulna ***m*** ulna (arm bone)
ultraviolet(te) ***adj*** ultraviolet
rayonnement ***m*** **ultraviolet** ultraviolet radiation
faire ***v*** **des séances d'ultraviolets** to have sunbed sessions
ultrason ***m*** ultrasound
ultrasonique ***adj*** ultrasonic
uncarthrose ***f*** neck vertebrae arthrosis
uncus ***m*** hook-formed bone
unité ***f*** ward; unit
urée ***f*** urea (nitrogenous compound in urine)
urémie ***f*** uraemia (raised blood level in nitrogeneous waste compounds)
uretère ***m*** ureter (urine canal from kidney to bladder)
urètre ***m*** urethra (urine discharge duct from the bladder)
urétéral(e) ***adj*** ureteral (of/ concerning the ureter)
urétral(e) ***adj*** urethral (of/ concerning the uretha)
urgence ***f*** emergency
service ***m*** **des urgences** casualty; casualty department
urgence ***f*** **médicale** medical emergency
uricémie ***f*** uric acid level in blood
urine ***f*** urine
urogénital(e) ***adj*** urogenital
urologie ***f*** urology (study of the urinary system)
urographie ***f*** **intraveineuse** intravenous X-ray of kidneys and urinary tracts
urticaire ***f*** urticaria; nettle rash; hives

usage *m* externe external use
(à) usage *m* unique single-use
utérus *m* uterus; womb
uvée *f* uveal tract (pigmented layer of the eye)

vaccin *m* vaccine
vaccin *m* anti-variolique small pox vaccine
vaccin *m* BCG BCG (Baccus Calmette-Guérin) vaccine
vaccin *m* contre la coqueluche pertussis vaccine; anti-whooping cough vaccine
vaccin *m* contre la rubéole rubella/German measles vaccine
vaccin *m* contre la diphtérie/le tétanos/la poliomyélite diphtheria/tetanus/poliomyelitis vaccine
vaccin *m* contre la grippe flu vaccine
vaccin *m* contre l'hépatite A hepatitis A vaccine
vaccin *m* contre l'hépatite B hepatitis B vaccine
vaccin *m* contre la tuberculose *f* TB vaccine
vaccination *f* vaccination
vacciner *v* to vaccinate
(se) faire vacciner *v* to have a vaccination
vache folle, maladie *f* de la mad cow disease
vagal(e) *adj* vagal (relating to vagus: a cranial nerve)
vagin *m* vagina
vaginal(e) *adj* vaginal
vaginité *f* inflammation of the vagina
vagotomie *f* surgery to the vagal nerve
vaisseau *m* (body) duct or canal
vaisseau *m* capillaire capillary (blood vessel type)
vaisseau *m* éclaté burst blood vessel
vaisseau *m* lymphatique lymph vessel
vaisseau *m* sanguin blood vessel (general term)
valériane *f* valerian (sedative)
valeurs *f* usuelles normal amounts
valga *adj* out-turned (limb)
valve *f* valve
valve *f* cardiaque heart valve
valvulaire *adj* concerning the heart valves

atteinte ***f*** **valvulaire** deterioration of heart valves
valvule ***f*** valve allowing blood flow in one direction
valvulopathie ***f*** heart valve disease
vaporisateur ***m*** spray; atomiser
vaporisateur ***m*** **d'eau thermale** spa water spray/atomiser
varice ***f*** varicose vein; varix
varicelle ***f*** chickenpox
varicocèle ***f*** expansion/widening of scrotum veins
variole ***f*** smallpox
vascularisé(e) ***adj*** vascular (containing blood vessels)
vase ***m*** **de lit; vase** ***m*** **de nuit** bedpan; chamberpot
vasectomie ***f*** vasectomy
vaseline® ***f*** vaseline®
vasoconstricteur ***m*** vasoconstrictor (agent causing constriction of blood vessels)
vasoconstricteur -trice ***adj*** causing constriction of blood vessels
vasoconstriction ***f*** vasoconstriction
vasodilatateur -trice ***adj*** vasodilating (causing dilatation of blood vessels)
vasodilatateur ***m*** **bronchique** product which aids dilation of bronchial tubes
vasodilatation ***f*** vasodilation
végétalien(ne) ***adj*** vegan
végétalisme ***m*** veganism
végétarien(ne) ***adj*** vegetarian
végétarisme ***m*** vegetarianism
végétations ***fpl*** **adénoïdes** adenoids
veine ***f*** vein
veine ***f*** **cave** vena cava (into the heart)
veine ***f*** **coronaire** coronary vein
veine ***f*** **jugulaire** jugular vein
veine ***f*** **porte** portal vein (to the liver)
veine ***f*** **pulmonaire** pulmonary vein
veineux -euse ***adj*** venous
retour ***m*** **veineux** blood return mechanism (to the heart)
vélo ***m*** **d'appartement** exercise bike
vélo ***m*** **d'intérieur** exercise bike
vénérien(ne) ***adj*** venereal

maladies ***fpl*** **vénériennes** venereal diseases
venin ***m*** venom
venimeux -euse ***adj*** venimous
ventilation ***f*** **artificielle/ assistée** artificial/assisted ventilation
ventilation ***f*** **respiratoire** respiratory ventilation
ventiler to ventilate (oxygenate the blood or admit/propel air into the lungs)
Ventoline® ***f*** Ventoline® (spray, syrup, or ampoule injection to counter asthma)
ventouse ***f*** cupping glass (applied to skin for counterirritation treatment)
ventral(e) ***adj*** relating to stomach
ventre ***m*** stomach; abdomen
avoir/prendre ***v*** **du ventre** to have/to be getting a paunch/ tummy
ventriculaire ***adj*** ventricular
insuffisance ***f*** **ventriculaire** ventricular insufficiency
ventricule ***m*** ventricle (body cavity or organ hollow)
ver ***m*** **solitaire** tapeworm
verge ***f*** penis
vergeture ***f*** stretch mark
vermifuge ***m*** vermifuge (expels intestinal worms)
verrue ***f*** wart
verrue ***f*** **plantaire** verruca
vertébral(e) ***adj*** vertebral
vertèbre ***f*** vertebra (*pl* -ae)
vertèbres ***fpl*** **cervicales** cervical vertebrae
vertèbres ***fpl*** **dorsales** dorsal vertebrae
vertèbres ***fpl*** **lombaires** lumbar vertebrae
vertébré ***m*** vertebrate
vertex ***m*** vertex (crown of the head)
vertige ***m*** dizziness; vertigo; giddiness
avoir ***v*** **des vertiges** to suffer from vertigo
vertigineux -euse ***ad*** vertiginous
vésical(e) ***adj*** concerning the bladder
vésication ***f*** vesicatory (eruption of blisters)
vésicatoire ***adj*** vesicatory
vésicule ***f*** vesicle (fluid-filled sac/cyst/blister)

vésicule *f* biliaire gall bladder

vésicules *fpl* génitales genital blisters/warts

vésicules *fpl* séminales seminal vesicles

vespéral(e) ***adj*** evening (of symptoms, etc.)

vessie *f* urinary bladder

vestibule ***m*** vestibule (channel/ chamber leading to another; part of the mouth outside the teeth)

vestibule *m* de l'oreille interne inner ear cavity

vibrations *fpl* vibrations

vibromasseur ***m*** vibrator

vieillesse *f* old age

vieillissement ***m*** ageing

vignette *f* medicine price sticker (used for social security reimbursement)

VIH ***m*** (abbreviation of **virus de l'immunodéficience *f* humaine)** see below

viol ***m*** rape

virémie *f* virus in the blood

virilisation *f* virilism (abnormal development of secondary male characteristics)

virologie *f* virology (study of viruses)

virus ***m*** virus

virus *m* de l'immunodéficience *f* humaine (VIH) human immunodeficiency virus (HIV)

visage ***m*** face

viscéral(e) ***adj*** visceral (relating to the body's principal interior organs)

viscères ***mpl*** viscera (organs)

vision *f* eyesight; vision

vision *f* double double vision

vitaliseur ***m*** vitaliser

visualiser to make visible (using med. equipment)

vitalité *f* vitality

vitamine *f* vitamin

comprimé *m* de vitamines vitamin tablet/pill

alimentation *f* riche/pauvre en vitamines food rich/poor in vitamins

vitaminé(e) ***adj*** with added vitamins

vitesse *f* de sédimentation globulaire red corpuscle sedimentation speed

vitiligo ***m*** vitiligo (skin depigmentation)

voie ***f*** duct; tract

voie ***f*** **biliaire** biliary duct

voie ***f*** **lacrymale** tear duct

par voie ***f*** **buccale/orale** orally

par voie ***f*** **nasale/rectale** through the nose/rectum (for administration of medicine)

par voie ***f*** **transvaginale** through the vagina

voies ***fpl*** **urinaires** urinary tract

voile ***m*** **au poumon** shadow on the lung

voiture ***f*** **pour handicapé** invalid car

volumétrie ***f*** measurement of volumes (in certain organs)

volumétrie ***f*** **vésicale prémictionnelle** measured amount of urine in full bladder

volvulus ***m*** volvulus; twisted (blocked) intestine

vomi ***m*** vomit

vomir ***v*** to vomit

vomissement ***m*** vomiting; vomit

voûte ***f*** **crânienne** dome of the skull; vault of the cranium

voûte ***f*** **palatine/du palais** roof of the mouth; hard palate

voûte ***f*** **plantaire** arch of the foot

VS ***f*** **(globulaire)** (abbrev. of **vitesse de sédimentation globulaire**) red corpuscle sedimentation speed

vue ***f*** eyesight; vision

vulve ***f*** vulva

vulvite ***f*** vulvitis (inflammation of the vulva)

vulvo-vaginite ***f*** inflammation of the vulva and vagina

water-closet ***m*** **(WC)** toilet; WC

Wolff-Parkinson-White, syndrome ***m*** **de** Wolff-Parkinson-White syndrome (sudden bursts of rapid heartbeats)

xanthome ***m*** xanthoma (skin disease)

yeux ***mpl*** eyes

yeux ***mpl*** **battus** dark or black rings under the eyes

zona *m* /herpès zoster *m*
shingles; herpes zosta

zona *m* ophtalmique shingles affecting eye and part of the face

zoonose *f* zoonosis (disease transmissible from animals to man)

zoopsie *f* zoopsy (hallucinations of seeing animals, associated with drugs and heavy drinking)

zostérien(ne) ***adj*** of/concerning shingles/herpes zosta

zygote *m* zygote (cell formed by union of two sexual reproduction cells)

zygomatique ***adj*** zygomatic

arcade *f* zygomatique zygomatic arch (prominent cheek bone)

os *m* zygomatique zygomatic bone

MEDICAL, HEALTH AND PHARMACY TERMS, PRODUCTS AND PLANTS

TERMES MEDICAUX, DE SANTE ET DE PHARMACIE, PRODUITS ET PLANTES

Comments and brief explanations, where considered appropriate, are in brackets after the English word or term. As with English translations in the previous section, there may be more than one translation in French. The French masculine *m* or feminine *f* gender is given after each noun.

2D ultrasound scan écho 2D *f*
2D X-rays imagerie *f* radiographie
3D electro-magnetic medical imagery exam remnographie *f* (using résonance *f* magnétique nucléaire)
3D medical imagery indicating how organs are functioning tépographie *f*
tomography (3D medical imagery/scanning) tomographie *f*
3D ultrasound scan échotomographie *f*

abasia (inability to walk) abasie *f*
abatement (of pain, fever); remission rémission *f*
abbreviations for antibiotic ATB, ATBT
abdomen; stomach abdomen *m*
abdominal cavity cavité *f* abdominale
abductor muscle abducteur *m*
abduction abduction *f*
abduction, with patient spreading limb away from body abduction *f* active
abduction, with doctor spreading limb away from body abduction *f* passive
abduction, with doctor pressing limb away from patient's body abduction *f* forcée
aberration (abnormal) aberration *f*
abnormality anomalie *f*; difformité *f*; malformation *f*
abortion avortement *m*
abortion (morning-after) pill pilule *f* abortive; pilule *f* du lendemain

ab(o)ulia (mental disorder with loss of willpower) aboulie *f*
ab(o)ulia sufferer aboulique *f*
abrasion écorchure *f*; érosion *f*
abscess abcès *m*
abscess of the liver abcès *m* du foie
abstention (from food) jeûne *m*
absorption absorption *f*
accommodation (automatic focussing function of the eyes) accommodation *f*
accumulation (for example of fatty deposits) accumulation *f*
ache douleur *f*
ache, to all over avoir *v* mal partout
aches and pains courbatures *f*
Achille's tendon tendon *m* d'Achille
aching douloureux –euse *adj*
achondroplasia (hereditary bone growth reduction) achondroplasie *f*
acidity acidité *f*
acidosis (blood with high acidity) acidose *f*
acne, childhood/adolescence acné *f* juvénile
acne spot bouton *m* d'acné *f*
acne cream antiacnéique *m*
acne, red; rosacea acné *f* rosacée; couperose *f*
acromegaly (growth hormone disorder causing gigantism) acromégalie *f*
acoumetry (hearing evaluation) acoumétrie *f*
active actif -ive *adj*
acupuncture acupuncture *f*
acute aigu(ë) *adj*
acuteness acuité *f*
Adam's apple pomme *f* d'Adam
adhesion (of two body parts), abnormal adhérence *f*
addiction (drug) dépendance *f*
addiction specialist addictologue *f*
Addison's disease (progressive anaemia, weakness and bronzing discolouration of skin) maladie *f* d'Addison; maladie bronzée *f*
adenitis (swelling of lymph nodes) adénite *f*
adenoids végétations *fpl* adénoïdes
adenoids, surgical removal of adénoïdectomie *f*

adduction (action of closing limbs to body) adduction *f*
adductor muscle adducteur *m*
adhesive plaster pansement *m* adhésif
adhesive tape, medical sparadrap *m*
adhesive tape, microporous sparadrap *m* microporeux
adiposity (excess body fat) adiposité *f*
adrenal gland (which secrets adrenaline) glande *f* surrénale
adrenalin adrénaline *f*
adolescence acne acné *f* juvénile
advise, to conseiller *v*
aerocoly (excessive air in large intestine) aérocolie *f*
aerogastria (excessive air in stomach) aérogastrie *f*
aerophagy (temporary excess air in stomach) aérophagie *f*
aerosol can bombe *f* aérosol
affected (by illness) atteint(e); pris(e) *adj*
afterbirth placenta *m*
after-care post-cure *f*; soins *m*
after-effect séquelle *f*
after-effect (consequences which can be sued for) séquelle *f* indemnisable
after-hours (duty) pharmacy pharmacie *f* de garde
after-sun lotion lotion *f* après-soleil
ageing vieillissement *m*
agglutination (clumping of bacteria, etc.) agglutination *f*
agglutinin (antibody etc. causing clumping) agglutinine *f*
AIDS (acquired immune deficiency syndrome) SIDA, sida *m* (Syndrome d'Immuno Déficience Acquise)
Aids screening dépistage *m* du sida *m*
air embolism embolie *f* gazeuse
air steriliser purificateur *m* d'air
agoraphobia agoraphobie *f*
albinism albinisme *m*
albumin (protein in egg-white, blood, milk) albumine *f*
albuminuria (abnormal protein count in urine) albuminurie *f*
alcohol alcool *m*

alcohol, amount of in the blood alcoolémie *f*; taux *m* d'alcoolémie

alcohol content; containing alcohol alcoolisé(e) *adj*

alcohol content, very low très peu alcoolisé(e)

alcohol (in blood) test contrôle *m* d'alcoolémie *f*

alcoholic (person) alcoolique *m/f*

alcoholic mania délire *m* alcoolique

alcoholism alcoolisme *m*

alcoholism, treatment for cure *f* de désintoxication

alcohol specialist alcoologue *m*

algae algues *fpl*

-algia (at end of words, denoting pain, e.g. in neuralgia) -algie

alimentary canal tube *m* digestif

alimentary canal, of/ conerning stromal(e) (*pl* -aux) *adj*

alimentary canal and windpipe, cross-over junction between carrefour *m* laryngé

alkaloid alcaloïde *m*

allergen allergène *m*

allergic allergique *adj*

allergy allergie *f*

allergy (to pollen, animal hairs, etc.) atopie *f*

allergy allievating antiallergique *adj*

allergy medicine (study and treatment) allergologie *f*

allergy-producing particles (in air) pneumallergène *m*

allergy test test *m* d'allergie *f*

allergy testing skin injection intradermo-réaction *f*

allopathy (conventional therapeutic method of treatment) allopathie *f*

alopecia (temporary, partial or complete hair loss) alopécie *f*; pelade *f*

alpha-blocker alphabloquant *m*

alternative medicine (therapy) médecine *f* alternative

alveolus (oxygen passage to the blood, in the lungs) alvéole *f* pulmonaire

Alzheimer's disease maladie *f* d'Alzheimer

ambulance ambulance *f*

ambulance service service *m* ambulancier

amenorrhoea (absence of menstrual periods) aménorrhée *f*

amoeba; ameba (tropical parasite) amibe *f*

amoeba/ameba infection amibiase *f*

ammonia ammoniac *m* (gas); ammoniaque *f* (liquid)

amnesia amnésie *f*

amnesia (after a stroke) amnésie *f* antérograde

amniocentis (amniotic fluid removal from the womb of pregnant mothers) amniocentèse *f*

amnion (innermost membrane enclosing the embryo) amnios *m*

amniotic (of innermost membrane) amniotique *adj*

amniotic (embryon) fluid liquide *m* amniotique

amount (dosage) dosage *m*

amphetamine (stimulant) amphétamine *f*

amputation amputation *f*

anabolic steroid anabolisant *m* stéroïdien

anaemia anémie *f*

anaesthesia (loss of body part sensitivity) anesthésie *f*

anaesthesia, epirudural (lower spinal cord) anesthésie *f* péridurale

anaesthesia, general anesthésie *f* générale

anaesthesia, local anesthésie *f* locale

anaesthesiology and post-operative reanimation anesthésiologie *f* et réanimation *f* chirurgicale

anaesthetic anesthésique *m* and *adj*

anaesthetist anesthésiste *m* and *f*

anal anal(e) *adj*

anal cleft raie *f* des fesses

anal pruritus (severe anal itching) prurit *m* anal

anal sphincter sphincter *m* anal

analgesia (absence/relief of pain) analgésie *f*

analgesic; anodyne analgésique *m* and *adj;* antidouleur *adj*

analgesic (pain reliever) antalgique *m*
analgesic medicine médicament *m* analgésique
anasarca (excess fluid in body tissues) anasarque *f*
anaphylactic shock choc *m* anaphylactique
(anatomical) wall paroi *f*
anatomical appendage appendice *m*
anatomical system appareil *m*
androgen (male hormone) androgène *m*
androgyne androgyne *m*
androsterone (male hormone) androstérone *f*
aneurism; aneurysm (abnormal swelling of artery) anévrisme *m;* anévrysme *m*
aneurysmal rupture (life-threatening) rupture *f* d'anévrisme
angelica plant angélique *f*
angina pectoris (impairment of blood vessels in heart) angine *f* de poitrine; angor *m*
angina pectoris sufferer angineux *m* -euse *f*
angioma (usually benign tumour formed by blood vessels, often a birthmark) angiome *m*
angiocardiography (X-ray examination of heart) angiocardographie *f*
angiography (X-ray of veins and arteries) angiographie *f*
anguish angoisse *f*
ankle cheville *f*
ankle bone (supporting the tibia) astragale *m*
ankylosing spondylitis (inflammation and stiffening of vertebrae) spondylarthrite *f* ankylosante
ankylosis (difficulty/inability to move a joint) ankylose *f*
anodyne analgésique *m* and *adj*
anomalous irrégulier -ère *adj*
anorexia (nervosa) anorexie *f* (mentale)
antacid antiacide *m*
anterior drawer sign of knee (tibia pulls forward or backward more than normal) tiroir *m* du genou

anthelmintic (drug or agent which destroys parasites) antihelminthique *m* and *adj*
anthrax (biological) disease maladie *f* du charbon *m*
antihistamine (product reducing/preventing allergies) antihistaminique *m*
antibacterial antibactérien(ne) *m/f* and *adj*
antibiotic antibiotique *m* and *adj*; érythromycine *f*
antibiotics, to be/put on être/mettre *v* sous antibiotiques *fpl*
antibiotic group closely related to penicillin céphalosporine *f*
antibiotic ointment pommade *f* antibiotique
antibiotics treatment antibiothérapie *f*
anti (blood) platelet aggregation antiagrégant *m* plaquettaire
antibody anticorps *m*
antibody causing clumping of bacteria agglutinine *f*
anticoagulant (treatment or substance) anticoagulant *m* ; anticoagulant(e) *adj*
anticonvulsant anticonvulsivant(e) *adj*
antidepressant antidépresseur *m*; remontant *m*
antidiphtheria serum sérum *m* antidiphthérique
antidiuretic antidiurétique *m*
antidote antidote *m*; contrepoison *m*
antagonists antagonistes *fpl*
antiemetic (used to combat side-effects of chemotherapy e.g. vomiting) antiémétiquc *m* and *adj*
anti-flu drug médicament *m* pour état grippal
antifungal antifongique *m* and *adj*
antigen antigène *m*
antihistamine (esp. to counter allergies) antihistaminique *m* and *adj*
anti-inflammatory anti-inflammatoire *adj*
antimitotic (chemical substance used in chemotherapy treatment) antimitotique *f*

anti-neoplastic (anticancer medicine) antinéoplasique *f*
antioxidant antioxydant *m*
antiperspirant déodorant *m* antisudoral
anti-pollution mask masque *m* anti-pollution
antipyretic (preventing/reducing fever) antipyrétique; fébrifuge *adj*
antipyretic drug or agent antipyrétique *m*; fébrifuge *m*
anti-rabies injection vaccination *f* antirabique
antiscorbutic (preventing/curing scurvy) antiscorbutique *adj*
antiseptic antiseptique *m* and *adj*; bleu de méthylène *m*
antiseptic compress compresse *f* antiseptique
antiseptic cream crème *f* antiseptique
antiseptics (use of) antisepsie *f*
antismoking patch/plaster timbre *m* transdermique (tabagisme *m*)
antispasmodic (medicine: also produced by the body) antispasmodique *m* and *adj*
antistasis (aids circulation) antistase *f*
antitetanus serum sérum *m* antitétanique
antitoxin antitoxine *f*
antiviral antiviral(e) *adj*
anuresis/anuria (kidney blockage) anurèse *f*; anurie *f*
anus anus *m*
anus infection irritation *f* anite
anus, artificial (temporary or permanent) anus *m* artificiel
aorta (main artery) aorte *f*
aorta rupture dissection *f* aortique
aorta X-ray aortographie *f*
aortic split (near stomach) bifurcation *f* aortique
apex (pointed tip/extremity of lung/heart, etc.) apex *m*
Apgar index (vitality rating of newborn baby) indice *m* d'Apgar
aphasia (total/partial loss of speech or understanding of speech due to brain disease/injury) aphasie *f*
aphonia (generally temporary, total voice loss) aphonie *f*

apnoea (involuntary holding of breath, especially during sleep) apnées *fpl* du sommeil

apoplectic fit attaque *f* d'apoplexie

appendicectomy/ appendectomy (appendix operation/removal) appendicectomie *f*

appendicitis appendicite *f*

appendicitis, acute appendicite *f* aiguë

appendicitis attack crise *f* d'appendicite *f*

appetite appétit *m*

appliance, medical appareil *m*

apply, to (ointment, etc.) mettre *v*; appliquer *v*

aquagym gymnastique *f* aquatique (aqua-gym)

aqueous humour/body (fluid between eye lens and cornea) humeur *f* aqueuse

arachnoid (middle membrane around brain and spinal cord) arachnoïde *f*

arch of the foot voûte *f* plantaire

arm bras *m*

arm, broken bras *m* cassé

armpit aisselle *f*

army medical officer médecin *m* militaire

arnica plant arnica *f*

aromatherapy (massage using oils and plant extracts) aromathérapie *f*

arrhythmia (irregular heartbeats) arythmie *f*

arterial embolism embolie *f* artérielle

arterial illnesses artériopathie *f*

arterial inflammation (due to diabetic condition) artériopathie *f* diabétique

arteriosclerosis (hardening of arteries) sclérose *f* artérielle; artériosclérose *f*

artery artère *f*

artery, inflammation of artérite *f*

artery, surgical repair of impaired angioplastie *f*

artery running along the radius artère *f* radiale

arthritis arthrite *f*

arthritis drug antiarthritique *m*

arthritis of the hip coxarthrose *f*

articular rheumatism (in the joints) rhumatisme *m* articulaire

articulary crepitation crépitation *f* articulaire

articulated leg jambe *f* articulée

articulation scan arthroscanner *m*

artificial insemination insémination *f* artificielle

artificial insemination by donor (AID) insémination *m* artificielle par donneur (IAD)

Asian flu grippe *f* asiatique

asbestos amiante *f*; asbeste *m* (less commonly used)

asbestosis (disease caused by long-term inhalation of asbestose particles) asbestose *f*

ascites (abnormal build-up of liquid in stomach) ascite *f*

ascorbic (acid vitamin in citrus fruits) ascorbique *adj* (acide)

ascorbic acid (Vitamin C) acide *m* ascorbique; vitamine C

asexual/sexless (person) asexué(e) *adj*

Asperger's syndrome (atypical personality development) syndrome *m* d'Asperger

asphyxia asphyxie *f*

asphyxiation étouffement *m*

aspirin acide *m* acétylsallcylique; aspirine *f*

aspirin, soluble aspirine *f* soluble

asthenia (weakness) asthénie *f*

asthma asthme *m*

asthma attack crise *f* d'asthme

asthma drug antiasthmatique *m* and *adj*

asthmatic asthmatique *adj*

astimagmatism (eye defect) astigmatisme *m*

astringent (of product which checks bleeding) astringent *m* and *adj*

ataxy/ataxia (loss of body movement control) ataxie *f*

atheroma (cholesterol build-up inside artery) athérome *m*

athlete's foot mycose *f* du pied; pied *m* d'athlète

atomiser vaporisateur *m*

atrium (upper heart cavity) orifice *f* de l'oreillette; atrium *m*

atrophy (dimunition in size or weight of an organ) atrophie *f*
attack (crisis; fit) crise *f*
attack, fever accès *m* de fièvre
attack, coughing accès *m* de toux
attributable imputable *adj*
audiogram (hearing test) audiogramme *m*
audiometer audiomètre *m*
auditory auditif -ve *adj*
auditory threshold seuil *m* auditif
auditory pain threshold: 120 decibels (DB) le seuil *m* auditif de douleur : 120 dB
aural acupuncture auriculothérapie *f*
auricle (of ear) pavillon *m* auriculaire; oreille *f* externe
auricle (of heart) oreillette *f* **left, right** gauche, droite
auricular fibrillation fibrillation *f* auriculaire (FA)
autism autisme *m*
autistic person autiste *m/f*
auto-blood transfusion (patient's own blood reserve is re-injected during an operation) autotransfusion *f*
autogenous (self-produced) autogène *adj*
autoclave (steam sterilisation apparatus) autoclave *m*
autoimmunisation, pathological autoimmunisation *f* pathologique
autoimmunisation, physiological autoimmunisation *f* physiologique
auto-intoxication auto-intoxication *f*
autolysis (milder way of saying 'suicide') autolyse *f*
automatic reflex (to doctor's reflex test) réflexe *m* ostéo-tendineux
automatism automatisme *m*
autopsy autopsie *f*
autoplasty (surgical operation using healthy tissue from the patient's body) autoplastie *f*
autotoxin (poison originating from patient's organism) autotoxine *f*
avian flu grippe *f* aviaire

awake, to keep/stay rester *v* éveillé
awareness (consciousness) conscience *f*
axis (second neck bone) axis *m*

baby cream crème *f* pour bébé
baby food alimentation *f* pour bébé
baby's dummy sucette *f*
baby lotion lait *m* de toilette pour bébé
baby powder talc *m*
baby shampoo shampooing/shampoing *m* pour bébé *m*
baby soap savon *m* pour bébé
baby wipes lingettes *fpl* pour bébé
bacillus (bacterial microbe) bacille *m*
back dos *m*
backache mal *m* de dos
backache (to have) avoir *v* mal aux reins
backbone épine *f* dorsale
back deformation déformation *f* dorsale
back rheumatism dosarthrose *f*
backrest appui-dos *m*
bactericide bactéricide *m* and *adj*
bacteriologist bactériologiste *m* and *f*
bacteriology bactériologie *f*
bacterium bactérie *f*
bad breath mauvaise haleine *f*; halitose *f*
balance an unbalanced diet, to supplémenter *v* une alimentation *f*
bald chauve *adj*
bald, to go se dégarnir *v*
baldness calvitie *f*
balm mélisse *f*; baume *m*
balneotherapy balnéothérapie *f*
balneotherapy mat (in the bath) matelas *m* de balnéothérapie
balneotherapy mat, remote-controlled matelas *m* de balnéothérapie télécommandé
Band-Aid ® plaster sparadrap *m*
bandage bandage *m*; bande *f*
bandage, chin mentonnière *f*
bandage, compressive pansement *m* compressif
bandage, crêpe bande *f* Velpeau ®

bandage, elastic support bande *f* de tissu élastique
bandage, plaster bande *f* plâtrée
bandage, small bandelette *f*
bandage, to bander *v*; panser *v*
barbiturate barbiturique *m*
barbiturate (amount in the blood) barbitémie *f*
barium enema (pre X-rays: coloscopy more usual) lavement *m* barite
barium sulphate and water meal (for stomach opacity prior to stomach X-rays) bouillie *f* de sulfate *m* de baryum
Basedow's disease (excessive hormone production following thyroid gland inflammation) maladie *f* de Basedow
basil basilic *m*
bathrooms; washrooms sanitaires *mpl*
battery (pacemaker, etc.) pile *f*
BCG (Baccus Calmette-Guérin) vaccine vaccin *m* BCG
beauty spot (mole) grain *m* de beauté
beauty spot, harmless naevus *m* simple
beauty spot, potentially cancerous naevus naevocellulaire *m*
bed lit *m*
bedpan bassin *m* hygiènique/de lit; vase *m* de lit
bedroom chambre *f* à coucher
bedsore escarre *f*
bed wetting, involuntary énusérie *f*; 'pipi au lit' *m*
bee sting piqûre d'abeille *f*
beginning of a course of treatment abord *m*
bella donna; deadly nightshade belladonna *f*
bends, the maladie *f* des caissons
benign bénin -igne *adj*
benign growth (often on a breast) adénofibrome *m*
benign tumour/growth adénome *m*
benzodiazepine (sedative group, incl. Valium ®) benzodiazepine *f* (abbrev. BZD)
beriberi béribéri *m*
best-before-date (foodstuffs) date limite de conservation *f*

beta blocker; beta blocking (controlling cardiac action) bétabloqueur *m;* bétabloquant *adj*

better general state of mental or physical well-being mieux-être *m*

bib bavoir *m*

biceps biceps *m*

biceps brachial muscle (arm) muscle *m* biceps brachial

biceps femoris muscle (thigh) muscle *m* biceps crural

bifocal spectacles lunettes *fpl* à double foyer

bigger, to get grossir *v*

bile bile *f*

bile amount in the blood bilirubinémie *f*

bile blockage cholestase *f*

bile duct canal *m* biliaire

bile duct from the liver, inflammation of angiocholite *f*

bile stone calcul *m* biliaire

bilharzia ('worms') bilharziose/schistomiase *f*

biliary colic colique *f* biliaire

biliary duct voie *f* biliaire

bilious bilieux -euse *adj*

bilious attack crise *f* de foie

bilirubin (one of bile's constituent substances) bilirubine *f*

bind, to (ligature) ligaturer *v*

biochemical laboratory laboratoire *m* biochimique

biochemistry biochimie *f*

biodegradability biodégradabilité *f*

biological test for hepatitis or AIDS virus ELISA (abbrev. from the English, enzyme-linked immunosorbent assay)

biological test in the anal area using sticky tape Scotch ® test *m*

biology biologie *f*

biopsy biopsie *f*

biopsy, sample (tissue, etc.) for fragment *m* biopsique

biorhythm biorythme *m*

birth, to give accoucher *v*

birth, to give (prematurely) accoucher *v* avant terme

birth, breech accouchement *m* par le siège

birth control contrôle *m* des naissances

birthmark angiome *m*; naevus *m* simple; tache *f* de naissance/de son

bistoury (surgical scalpel) bistouri *m*

bite morsure *f*

bite, insect piqûre *f*

blepharitis (eyelid inflammation) blépharite *f*

(to be) black and blue all over/covered in bruises (être) *v* tout meurtri *adj*

blackcurrant cassis *m*

black eye œil *m* poché; œil *m* au beurre noir

blackhead comédon *m*; point *m* noir

blackout (pass out) évanouissement *m*; syncope *f*

blackout, to tomber *v* en syncope

bladder vessie *f*

bladder, of the vésical(e) (*p.* -aux) *adj*

bladder inflammation; cystitis cystite *f*

bleed, to saigner *v*

bleeding (blood letting) saignée *f*

bleeding saignement *m*

bleeding, heavy pertes *fpl* de sang

bleeding time before coagulation temps *m* de saignement

blind man/woman aveugle *m/f*

blindness cécité *f*

blind spot (anatomical) tache *f* aveugle

blinking (reaction to approaching objects) réflexe *m* palpébral

blinking, continual and involuntary papillotage *m*

blister ampoule *f*; cloque *f*

full of blisters couvert(e) *adj* d'ampoules *fpl*

blister (medical); vesicle ampoule *f*; vésicule *f*

blister, to cloquer

blister(s) eruption vésication *f*

blister plaster pansement *m* pour ampoule

blistering (skin condition) (état *m*) bulleux -euse *adj*

bloating ballonnement *m*

blob (of gel) noisette *f* (de gel)

blockage blocage *m*; obstruction *f*

blockage, intestinal occlusion *f* intestinale

blockage, mental blocage (mental)

block, memory blocage *m* (mental)

blocked/paralysed joints (in flexed position) flessum/ flexum *m*

blood sang *m*

blood, abnormal fat level in dyslipidémie *f*/ dyslipémie *f*

blood, contaminated sang *m* contaminé

blood, flow of flux *m* de sang

blood, inflammation/ overheating of échauffement *m*

blood acidity increase (diabetes complication) acidocétose *f*

blood air components gaz *m* du sang

blood bank banque *f* de sang

blood blister pinçon *m*

blood cell cellule *f* sanguine

blood circulation bypassing main artery or vein circulation *f* collatérale

blood circulation, poor (with 'blue' extremities) acrocyanose *f*

blood circulation, its disease and treatment angiologie *f*

blood circulation, external pumps/tubes maintaining (during open-heart surgery) circulation *f* extra-corporelle (CEC)

blood clot caillot *m*

blood clot elimination (with an enzyme) fibrinoylise *f*

blood clotting agent agent *m* coagulant de sang

blood coagulation agent facteur *m* de la coagulation

blood coagulation substance *f* prothrombine

blood coagulation, type of liquid produced after hématique *adj*

blood corpuscle globule *m* sanguin

blood count numération *f* globulaire

blood count(s)/test(s) bilan(s) *m* sanguin(s)

blood count normal amounts (ranges shown on blood-test results) valeurs usuelles *fpl*

blood derivatives (from blood donors) dérivés *mpl* du sang; produits *mpl* sanguins

blood donation don *m* du sang

blood group/type groupe *m* sanguin

blood plasma plasma *m* sanguin

blood pocket (resulting from bruise) kyste *m* hématique

blood poisoning empoisonnement *m* du sang; toxémie *f*

blood pressure pression *f* artérielle; tension *f* artérielle; tension *f*

blood pressure, high hypertension *f*

to suffer from high blood pressure souffrir *v* d'hypertension

blood pressure, increase in (during pregnancy) toxémie *f*

blood pressure, low hypotension *f*

blood pressure, lowered tension *f* baissée

blood pressure measurement instrument sphygmomanomètre *m*

blood pressure, raised tension *f* montée

blood pressure, sudden drop in malaise *m* vasovagal

blood pressure, to check vérifier *v* la tension

blood pressure, to take prendre *v* la tension

blood product (red corpuscles, platelets) produit *m* sanguin

blood return (to the heart) mechanism retour *m* veineux

blood reflux (from liver to jugular vein) reflux *m* hépato-jugulaire

blood sample prélèvement *m* de sang; prise *f* de sang

blood serum (concerning) sérique *adj*

blood-flow speed measurement test using ultrasound vélocimétrie doppler *f*

blood-flow measurement combining ultrasound echo and ultrasound scan measurement (graphie) doppler *m*

blood-shot eyes yeux *mpl* injectés de sang

blood smear frottis *m* sanguin

blood specialist; haematologist hématologue *m/f*

blood substance which increases with muscle disorder créatine phosphokanise *f* (CPK)

blood substances requiring identification prior to transfusion(s) agglutinines *fpl* irrégulières

blood sugar level sucre *m* dans le sang

blood-system vascular disease (angeitis) angéite *f*

blood test/analysis analyse *f* de sang; examen *m* du sang

blood test measuring rate of coagulation temps *m* de Quick, temps *m* de quinine

blood test for ion count ionogramme *m*

blood test laboratory laboratoire *m* d'analyses *fpl* médicales

blood transfusion transfusion *f* sanguine

blood vessel vaisseau *m* sanguin

blood vessel, burst vaisseau *m* éclaté

blood vessels, drug causing dilatation of; minoxidil minoxidil *m*

blood vessel diseases (general term) angiopathie *f*

blood virus count charge *f* virale

blood with high acidity; acidosis acidose *f*

blotchy (face) masque *m* ecchymotique

'blue' baby (with congenital heart or blood circulation condition) enfant 'bleu' *m*

'blue' disease; congenital cyanosis (oxygen-deficient blood) cyanose *f*; maladie *f* bleue

body corps *m*

body, foreign corps *m* étranger

body, yellow (hormone-secreting structure in ovary) corps *m* jaune

body, vitreous (the eye) corps *m* vitré

body, area of région *f*

body channel/passage méat *m*

body duct/canal vaisseau *m*
body fat, excess adiposité *f*
body fat increase (under skin) lipomatose *f*
body hair poil *m*
body lotion lait *m* pour le corps
body mass index (BMI) indice *m* de masse *f* corporelle (IMC) (see indice de masse corporelle in French-English section for calculation example and weight categories)
body measurements and weight biométrie *f*
body's natural defence system réaction *f* immunitaire
body organ collapse aplasie *f*
body susceptible to illness terrain *m*
body tone tonicité *f*
boil clou *m*; furoncle *m*
boil, to bouillir *v*
bolster (neck, head, back support) traversin *m* bolus; (pellet/capsule) bol *m*
bone os *m*, os (*pl*)
bone cancer ostéosarcome *m*
bone crepitation crépitation *f* osseuse
bone decay carie *f*
bone density increase condensation *f* d'un os
bone density and calcium content measurement ostéodensitométrie *f*
bone development time graph compared to child's real age âge *m* osseux
bone fracture, internal fixation of (using metal nails, screws, plates) ostéosynthèse *f*
bone fragment (following necrosis) séquestre *m*
bone growth reduction, hereditary; achondroplasia achondroplasie *f*
bone inflammation or bone disease; osteitis ostéite *f*
bone marrow moelle *f* osseuse
bone marrow or bone or inflammation; osteomyelitis ostéomyélite *f*
bone marrow transplant greffe *f* de moelle *f* osseuse
bone socket cavité *f* articulaire
bone socket receiving another bone (esp. socket receiving top of thigh bone) cotyle *f*
bone splinter esquille *f*

bone tissue tissu *m* osseux

bone formation (abnormal) on top of normally developed bone exostose *f*

bone tumour (harmless) ostéome *m*

bony osseux -euse *adj*

booster seat (toilets) siège *m* rehausseur

booster shot/injection/jab piqûre *f*; piqûre *f* de rappel

booster (tonic) remontant *m*

borage plant bourrache *f* officinale

boss-eyed/cross-eyed, to be avoir *v* les yeux *m* qui se croisent *v*

bottle, small flacon *m*

bottle with measure for drops, small flacon *m* doseur

bottle feed, to (milk) allaiter *v* au biberon *m*; nourrir *v* au biberon *m*

bottle feeding allaitement *m* artificiel

botulism (serious food poisoning through poor food conservation) botulisme *m*

bout/burst (sudden attack of) accès *m*

bowel (small intestine) intestin *m* grêle

bowel irritation disorder colopathie *f* fonctionnelle

bowels intestins *mpl*

bowels and bladder, correct functioning of; continence continence *f*

bow-legged jambes arquées *fpl*

brace appareil *m* orthopédique

brace, metal (for broken bone) fixateur *m* externe

bradycardia (abnormally slow pulse) bradycardie *f*

brain cerveau *m*

brain activity examination électroencéphalographe *m*

brain activity recording (monitoring) électroencéphalogramme *m*

brain damage lésion *f* cérébrale

brain-dead coma dépassé *m*

brain death mort *f* cérébrale

brain fever fièvre *f* cérébrale

brain fissure, lateral scissure *f* latérale/de Sylvius

brain fissure, longitudinal scissure *f* interhémisphérique

brain membrane (tent-like membrane adjacent to cerebellum) tente *f*
brain or nerve tumour gliome *m*
brain tumour astrocytome *f*
break, to casser *v*
breast sein *m*; poitrine *f*
breast and bottle feeding allaitement *m* mixte
breast cancer cancer *m* du sein
breast enlargement hypertrophie *f* mammaire
breast-feed a baby, to donner à téter *v* à un bébé
breast-feeding allaitement *m* maternel
breast illnesses, study and treatment of sénologie *f*
breast inflammation; mastitis mastite *f*
breast prosthesis prothèse *f* mammaire
breast specialist sénologue *m*
breast surgery, cosmetic plastie *f* mammaire; mammoplastie *f*
breath, to take a deep respirer *v* bien fort
breathalyser test Alcootest ® *m*
breathalyse, to (using device) faire subir *v* un Alcootest ®
breathe, to respirer *v*
breathe in, to inhaler *v*
breathe with difficulty, to respirer *v* avec difficulté
breathe in respirez *imp*
breathing respiration *f*
breathing, abnormal rubbing noise accompanying frottement *m* pleural
breathing, person with good eupnéïque *m/f*
breathing (through the mouth/nose) respiration *f* (buccale/nasale) *adj*
breathing-aid medicine eupnéïque *f*
breathing-difficulty sufferer dyspnéique *m* and *f*
breathing exercises kinésithérapie *f* respiratoire
breathing exercise which swells chest ampliation *f* thoracique
breathing in inspiration *f*
breathing-in, difficulty dyspnée *f* inspiratoire
breathing inability (when lying down) orthopnée *f*

breathing insufficiency hypopnée *f*

breathing insufficiency sufferer insuffisant(e) *m/f* respiratoire

breathing mask masque *m* respiratoire

breathing, rapid (possibly abnormal) polypnée *f*

breathing rate fréquence *f* respiratoire

breathing rate, abnormally slow bradypnée *f*

breathing tube, insertion of into windpipe intubation *f* trachéale; trachéotomie *f*

breathlessness étouffement *m*

breech position (for childbirth) présentation *f* par le siège

complete/full breech position siège *m* complet

bring about, to (an illness) engendrer *v*

Bright's disease (chronic kidney disease) néphrose *f*

broken (limb) cassé *adj*

bronchial tube bronche *f*

bronchial tubes, contraction of bronchospasme *f*

bronchial tubes, widening of bronchectasie *f*

bronchial tube dilation dilatation *f* des bronches *f*

bronchial tube dilatation aid (product) vasodilateur *m* bronchique

bronchialitis (potentially serious infection in babies) bronchiolite *f*

bronchioles (small tubes off bronchial tubes) bronchioles *fpl*

bronchitis bronchite *f*

bronchodilator (treats asthma) bronchodilateur *m*

brucellosis brucellose *f*

bruise bleu *m*; contusion *f*; ecchymose *f*; hématome *m*

bruise, to contusionner *v*; meurtrir *v*

bruised contusionné(e) *adj*; meurtri(e) *adj*; ecchymotique *adj*

bruxism (clenching/grinding of teeth) mâchonnement *m*

buccal (concerning the mouth) buccal(e) *adj*

buffer (chemical agent countering addition of acid or alkali) tampon *m*
bulbous-shaped organ or organ part bulbe *m*
bulging (eyes) saillant(e) *adj*
bulimia boulimie *f*
build, of slight/medium/stout de faible/moyenne/forte corpulence *f*
build up one's health, to accroître *v* son capital santé
bump bosse *f*
bunion oignon *m*
burdock (used for cough syrup) bardane *f*
burn brûlure *f*
burn, first/second/third degree brûlure *f* du premier/deuxième/troisième degré
burn, to brûler *v*
burp éructation *f*
bursitis (inflammation of a bursa/fluid-filled sac) bursite *f*; hygroma *m*
burst, to (blister, blood vessel) éclater *v*; percer *v*
burst an abscess, to crever *v* un abcès
burst blood vessel vaisseau *m* éclaté
buttock fesse *f*
buzzing (imaginary) in the ears acouphène *m*
buzzing/ringing in the ears bourdonnement *m* d'oreilles
bypass operation/surgery pontage *m*
by-product dérivé *m*

cæcum (first part of large intestine) cæcum *m*
Caesarean birth césarienne *f*
calamine calamine *f*
calamine lotion lotion *f* calmante à la calamine
calcaneum (heel bone) calcanéum *m*
calcaneum, pointed bone abnormality below the épine *f* calcanéenne
calcaneum, of the calcanéen(e) *adj*
calcareous sedimentation (of tissue/organ, blocking their functionning) dégénérescence *f* calcaire
calcareous stones (in the body) concrétion *f* calcaire

calcification in small blocked vein phlébolithe *m*
calcium calcium *m*
calcium amount in blood calcémie *f*
calcium content/level and bone density measurement ostéodensitométrie *f*
calcium blocker treating high blood pressure inhibiteur *m* calcique
calcium-depositing (illness) calcifiant(e) *adj*
calcium level in bone(s) densité *f* osseuse; minéralisation *f*
calcium level in bones measurement densitométrie *f* osseuse
calcium loss in bones, abnormal; demineralisation déminéralisation *f*
calcification calcification *f*
calculous (stony) pierreux -euse *adj*
calculus (stone) calcul *m*
calf (muscle) mollet *m*
callisthenics (body work-out gym) gymnastique *f* suédoise
callous (skin) calleux –euse *adj*
callus cal *m*; callosité *f*; durillon *m*
calm tranquille *adj*
canal canal *m*
cancer cancer *m*
cancer, bone ostéosarcome *m*
cancer, breast cancer *m* du sein
cancer, cervical cancer *m* du col de l'utérus
cancer specialist cancérologue *m*; oncologue *m*
cancer and oncology (tumours) medicine, study/ practice of cancérologie *f*, oncologie *f*
cancer of the liver cancer *m* du foie
cancer patient cancéreux –euse *m/f*
cancer producing cancérigène *adj*
cancer phobia cancérophobie *f*
cancer throughout the body cancer *m* généralisé
cancer ward service *m* de cancer
cancerous cancéreux –euse *adj*
cancerous growth processus *m* cancéreux
cancerous tumour/growth adénocarcinome *m*

cancerous growth (early stages) in the cervix dysplasie *f* du col de l'utérus

Candida albicans (fungus that causes thrush) candida albicans *m*

candidosis (see also thrush) candidose *f*; moniliase *f*

canine (tooth) canine *f*

capillary capillaire *m*

capillary (blood vessel) vaisseau *m* capillaire

capping (of tooth) couronne *f* dentaire

capsule capsule *f*

carbohydrate glucide *m*; hydrate *m* de carbone

carbohydrate glucidique *adj*

carbon monoxide oxyde de carbone *m*; monoxyde de carbone *m*

carbuncle(s) anthrax *m*

carcinoma (cancers of skin, digestive tract and lung) carcinome *m*

cardiac cardiaque *adj*

cardiac arrest arrêt *m* cardiaque

cardiac block (pulse blockage) bloc *m* cardiaque

cardiac insufficiency sufferer; 'cardiac' insuffisant(e) *m/f* cardiaque

cardiac massage massage *m* cardiaque

cardiac murmur souffle *m* cardiaque

cardiac shock choc *m* cardiogènique

cardiogram (record of heart muscle activity) cardiogramme *m*

cardiograph (instrument which measures heart muscle activity) cardiographe *m*

cardiologist (heart and blood circulation specialist) cardiologue *m*

cardiology (study/treatment of heart and blood circulation) cardiologie *f*

cardiomyopathy (**heart muscle disease)** cardiomyopathie *f*

cardiovascular cardio-vasculaire *adj*

cardiovascular disease maladie *f* cardio-vasculaire

cardiovascular system système *m* cardio-vasculaire

carditis (inflammation of heart membranes) cardite *f*

care soins *mpl*

carotene/carotin (Vitamin A orange or red pigment) carotène *m*

carotid (either of two arteries from heart to neck and head) carotide *f*

carotid sinusitis sinus *m* carotidien

carpal canal (duct containing tendons linked to finger bones) canal *m* carpien

carpus -i (*pl*) (wrist bone(s)) carpe *m*; os *m* du carpe

carrier (contagious germs, viruses) porteur *m* -euse *f*

carrier (contagiousgerms, viruses), not in themselves affected porteur *m* –euse *f* sain(e)

cartilage cartilage *m*

cartilage disorders chondropathie *f*

case cas *m*

castor oil huile *f* de ricin

castration castration *f*

casualty/casualty department service *m* des urgences

catalepsy catalepsie *f*

catalyst facteur *m* déclenchant

cataplasm cataplasme *m*

cataract cataracte *f*

catarrh catarrhe *m*

catch a chill, to attraper *v* un coup de froid; attraper *v* un refroidissement *m*

catch a cold, to attraper *v* un coup de froid; prendre *v* froid

catgut catgut *m*

cathartic cathartique *m* and *adj*

catheter cathéter *m*; sonde *f* creuse; sonde *f* à canal central

catheterisation (using catheter to inject into veins) cathétérisme *m*

catheterisation (probe) sondage *m*

cauterisation cautérisation *f*

cauterisation (with electrically heated instrument) cautère *m*

cauterise, to cautériser *v*

cavity (anatomy) cavité *f*; fosse *f*

cavity, abnormal (in an organ) diverticule *m*

cell cellule *f*

cell samples (for analysis) cytoponction *f*

cellulite; cellulitis (inflammation of cell tissue) cellulite *f*

central nervous system (brain, spinal cord) système *m* nerveux central

cephalagia (headache) céphalée *f*; mal *m* de tête

cerebellum (back of the brain) cervelet *m*

cerebral cérébral(e) *adj*

cerebral cotex (outer part of brain) cortex *m* cérébral

cerebral embolism embolie *f* cérébrale

cerebral palsy paralysie *f* cérébrale

cerebrospinal céphalo-rachidien –ienne *adj*

cerebrospinal fluid liquide *m* cérébrospinal

cervical (womb) cancer cancer *m* du col de l'utérus

cervical cerclage (surgical procedure performed during pregnancy where cervix is sewn closed) cerclage *m* du col de l'utérus

cervical mucus glaire *f* cervicale

cervical screening examen *m* endocervical

cervical smear frottis *m* cervovaginal (FV)

cervical vertebrae vertèbres *fpl* cervicales

cervix (neck of the womb) col *m* de l'utérus

cervix, surgical removal of part of conisation *f*

chain smoker tabagique *m/f*, fumeur -euse

chalazion (small abscess in/on eyelid) chalazion *m*

chamber pot pot *m* de chambre

chancre chancre *m* syphilitique

chancroid; soft chancre (VD groin ulcer) chancre *m* mou; chancrelle *f*

changing (mood, condition) labile *adj*

chap, to crevasser *v*

chapped, to become se crevasser *v*

chapped, badly (hands/knees) plein(e)s *adj* de gerçures

chapping gerçure *f*

characteristically specific (symptom) spécifique *adj*

charcoal/carbon, activated (for adsorptive properties) charbon *m* activé

cheek joue *f*

cheekbone pommette *f*

chemist pharmacien(ne) *m/f*

chemist's pharmacie *f*

chemotherapy chimiothérapie *f*; (abbrev.) chimio *f*

chest pectoral *m*

chest/ribs, parietal pain in the (not the heart) douleur *f* pariétocostale

chest expander extenseur *m*

chew, to mâchonner *v*

chewable tablet cachet *m* à croquer

chewing mâchonnement *m*; mastication *f*

chickenpox varicelle *f*

chilblain engelure *f*

child and adolescent psychiatry psychiatrie *f* de l'enfant *m* et de l'adolescent *m*

child surgery, practice/study of médecine *f* de chirurgie *f* infantile

childbirth (in confinement) en couches

childbirth; delivery accouchement *m*

childbirth, difficulty in dystocie *f*

childbirth, difficult type of dystocique *adj*

childbirth, easy (minimum medical assistance) accouchement *m* spontané

childbirth, full-term accouchement *m* à terme

childbirth, head-presentation position during présentation *f* par la tête

childbirth contractions contractions *fpl* utérines

childbirth labour travail *m*

childbirth, period immediately following; post-partum post-partum *m*

childhood disease/complaint maladie *f* infantile

child's height-weight growth/development chart développement *m* staturo-pondéral

chill coup de froid *m*; refroidissement *m*

chill (shiver) frisson *m*

chin menton *m*

chin bandage mentonnière *f*
chiropodist pédicure *m/f*
chiropody podologie *f*; soins *mpl* de pédicure/du pied
chiropractor (usually not a doctor) chiropracteur *m*
chiropractic (manipulation of the joints) chiropractie *f*
chlamidia (small parasitic bacterium) chlamydia *f*
chloasma (dark patches on face occurring sometimes in pregnancy) masque *m* de grossesse
chloral hydrate (sedative) hydrate *m* de chloral
choking suffocation *f*
choking fits, to have avoir *v* des suffocations *fpl*
cholera choléra *m*
cholesterol cholestérol *m*
cholesterol, abnormal amount of in blood hypercholestérolémie *f*
cholesterol (anti-) medicines/ drugs statines *fpl*
cholesterol count in the blood cholestérolémie *f*
cholesterol level (per litre of blood) taux *m* de cholestérol total
cholesterol build-up inside artery; atheroma athérome *m*
cholycystectomy (surgical removal of the gall bladder) cholécystectomie *f*
chorion (outermost membrane around an embryo) chorion *m*
chromosome chromosome *m*
chromosomal aberration aberration *f* chromosomique
chronic chronique *adj*
chronic bronchopneumonia broncho-pneumopathie *f* chronique obstructive (BPCO)
chronic disease maladie *f* chronique
chronic lupus erythematis (ulcerous skin disease) lupus *m* érythémateux chronique
choroiditis (inflammation of eye membrane) choroïdite *f*
chyle (whitish digestive fluid in small intestine) chyle *m*
cigarette burn brûlure *f* de cigarette

circulation of the blood circulation *f* sanguine

circumcision circoncision *f*; posthectomie *f*

cirrhosis of the liver cirrhose *f* du foie

citric acid acide *m* citrique

claustrophobia claustrophobie *f*

clavicle clavicule *f*

cleanliness (for good health) hygiènisme *m*

cleansing of wound/cut, removing any immediately surrounding dead skin parage *m*

cleansing lotion lotion *f* de toilette

cleansing milk lait *m* de toilette

clear, to (nose, throat, chest, etc.) dégager *v*

clear one's throat, to se racler *v* la gorge

cleft palate palais *m* fendu

clenching (of teeth) mâchonnement *m*

clinical examination (doctor's simple examination) examen *m* clinique

clinical death (by observation of patient's condition) mort *f* clinique

clinical picture (observations) tableau *m* clinique

clinical sign signe *m* clinique

clitoris clitoris *m*

clone clone *m*

closed (stuck) eyelid occlusion *f* palpébrale

club foot pied *m* bot

clumping (of bacteria etc.); agglutination agglutination *f*

coagulant coagulant *m*

coagulation coagulation *f*

coagulation, blood test measuring rate of temps *m* de Quick; temps *m* de coagulation

coated tablet comprimé *m* pelliculé

cobalt therapy unit bombe *f* au cobalt

coccyx coccyx *m*

cochlea (snail-shaped cavity inside ear) limaçon *m* osseux; cochlée *f*

codeine (pain killer) codéine *f*

cod-liver oil huile *f* de foie de morue

cold coup *m* de froid; rhume *m*
cold sore (lip/lip area) bouton *m* de fièvre; herpès *m* de la lèvre
cold sores (mouth area) herpès *m* buccal
colibacillosis (bacterial infection in large intestine) colibacillose *f*
colic colique *f* (abbrev. of douleur *f* colique)
colic, in the jaw and cheek colique *f* salivaire
colitis (inflammation of the colon) colite *f*
collagen (major structural protein) collagène *m* and *adj*
collar-bone clavicule *f*
Colles' arm fracture; (lower radius) fracture *f* de Pouteau-Colles
colon (major part of large intestine) côlon *m*
colonic colonique *adj*
colonise, to (be overrun by/ infested by) coloniser *v*
coloscopy (examination by optic fibres inside the colon) coloscopie *f*
colostomy (surgical operation to replace part of the colon, bypassing the anus) colostomie *f*
colostrum (first post-natal breast secretion) colostrum *m*
colour blind daltonien(ne) *adj*
colour-blind person daltonien(ne) *m/f*
colour blindness daltonisme *m*
colposcopy (vaginal and neck of the womb examination) colposcopie *f*
coma coma *m*
coma, deep coma *m* profond
coma, fall into a tomber dans le coma *m*
Glasgow Coma Scale barème *m* de Glasgow
comatose with good response coma *m* vigile
comatose with poor response coma *m* léger
comb peigne *m*
comb, to (oneself) se peigner *v*
comb, fine-tooth (for removeing lice) peigne *m* à poux
comedogenic (blocks the pores) comédogène *adj*

compatability compatibilité *f*

compensation (helpful/ curative physiological modification or psychological reaction) compensation *f*

complaint doléance *f*

complementary foodstuff(s) (for balanced nutrition) complément *m* alimentaire

complex (slow) sugars sucres *mpl* lents

complications complications *fpl*

complications following a physical/mental trauma post-traumatique *adj*

compress compresse *f*

compress, hot/cold compresse *f* 'physiopack'

compress, to compresser *v*

compression of the spinal column tassement *m* de la colonne verticale

compressive compressif –ive *adj*

compressive bandage pansement *m* compressif

compulsive eating boulimie *f*

compulsive eater boulimique *f*

concentration, lack of (in person) désorientation *f* d'un malade

conception conception *f*

concretion (stony mass formed in body) concrétion *f*

concussed commotioné(e) *adj*

concussion commotion *f* cérébrale

terminally ill condamné(e) *adj*

condom préservatif *m*

conduction (of blood) conduction *f*

confine, to (someone to a mental hospital/institution) interner *v*

confinement internement *m*

confinement, in (childbirth) en couches *fpl*

confinement to bed alitement *m*

congenital congenital(e) *adj*

congenital diseases affections *fpl* congénitales

congenital malformation of organ transposition *f*

congenital testicle complaint (felt in stomach) cryptorchidie *f*

congestion congestion *f*

congestion of the lungs congestion *f* pulmonaire
conjunctivitis conjonctivite *f*
connective tissue tissu *m* conjonctif
consanguinity consanguinité *f*
consciousness conscience *f*; connaissance *f*
consciousness, to lose perdre *v* conscience
consciousness, to regain reprendre *v* conscience
consent of patient/family (after explanation) consentement *m* ('éclairé')
conservation stipulations conditions *fpl* de conservation
constipation constipation *f*; échauffement *m* du ventre; stase *f* stercorale
constipated constipé(e) *adj*
constipated (person) constipé(e) *m/f*
constitution constitution *f*
consultant (hospital) médecin *m* d'hôpital
contact allergy allergie *f* de contact
contact lenses lentilles *f* de contact
contagion/contagiousness contagion *f*
contagious disease maladie *f* contagieuse
contagious bird disease psittacose *f*
contain, to (an infection) circonscrire *v* une infection
contaminate, to (blood, etc.) contaminer *v*
contaminated contaminé(e) *adj*
contamination contamination *f*
continence continence *f*
contraception contraception *f*
contraceptive (all types) contraceptif *m*
contraceptive pill pilule *f* (informal); pilule *f* contraceptive
contraction (muscle, retina) rétrécissement *m*
contraindication (of medicine) contre-indication *f*
convalescence convalescence *f*
copper cuivre *m*
cord cordon *m*
cord, spinal cordon *m* médullaire
cord, umbilical cordon *m* ombilical

corn cor *m*; hyperkératose (not necessarily on the toes)

corn plaster emplâtre *m* pour les cors

cornea cornée *f*

cornea graft kératoplastie *f*

cornea, inflammation of; keratitis kératite *f*

cornea, thickening of kératose *f*

coronary coronaire *adj*

coronary bypass operation pontage *m* coronarien

coronary heart disease maladie *f* coronarienne

coronary thrombosis thrombose *f* coronarienne; infarctus *m* du myocarde

coronary vein veine *f* coronaire

corpulence corpulence *f*

correct, to (vision, etc) corriger

corrective vision glasses (spectacles) lunettes *fpl* de vue

cortex (external part of an organ) cortex *m*

corticoid (substance produced by gland above the kidney); medicinal group treating inflammations and allergies corticoïde *m*

corticoid course of treatment corticothérapie *f*

cortisone cortisone *f*

coryza (head cold) coryza *m*

cosmetic surgery chirurgie *f* esthétique

cot death (unexplained) mort *f* subite (inexpliquée) du nourisson

cotton wool ouate *f* hydrophile

couch grass chiendent *m*

cough/coughing toux *f*

cough, dry toux *f* sèche

cough, hard (with larynx inflammation) croup *m*

cough, loose toux *f* grasse

cough, nervous toux *f* nerveuse

cough, smoker's toux *f* de fumeur

cough, to tousser *v*

coughing attack accès de toux *m*

cough drop/lozenge/pastille pastille *f* pour la toux

coughing fit crise *f* de toux

cough mixture; cough syrup antitussif *m*; sirop *m* pectoral/ sirop *m* pour la toux

cough mixture (to break up fluid in bronchial tubes) fluidifiants *mpl* bronchiques
counteract, to neutraliser *v*
counterirritation treatment révulsion *f*
course (of treatment) cure *f*
crack (skin) gerçure *f*
cramp contraction *f* musculaire
cramp in the calf crampe *f* au mollet
cranial nerve nerf *m* crânien
cranium crâne *m*
crazy fou *m*/folle *f adj*
crazy (man/woman) fou *m*/folle *f*
cream crème *f*
cream (pharmaceutical/ cosmetic) pâte *f*
creamy onctueux –euse *adj*
creatine (protein metabolism produced in muscles) créatine *f*
creatine amount in the blood créatinémie *f*
crêpe bandage bande *f* Velpeau ®
crêpe glove (for body scrub) gant *m* de crêpe
crepitation (crackling/ rattling noise) crépitation *f*; grésillement *m*
crepitation, articulary crépitation *f* articulaire
crepitation, bone crépitation *f* osseuse
crepitation, lung crépitation *f* pulmonaire
cretinism crétinisme *m*
Creutzfeld-Jakob disease maladie *f* de Creutzfeld-Jakob
Crohn's disease (chronic intestinal inflammation) maladie *f* de Crohn; iléite *f* régionale
cross-eyed/boss-eyed, to be avoir *v* les yeux qui se croisent *v*
cross-section coupe *f* transversale
crotch entre les jambes *f*
croup (larynx inflammation and hard cough) croup *m*
croup, spasmodic faux croup *m*
crown (of tooth) couronne *f*
crown (of the head) vertex *m*
crutch béquille *f*
crutch, underarm béquille *f* commune

crutch, forearm béquille *f* d'avant-bras

crying fit, to have a avoir *v* une crise de larmes

cryotherapy (low-temperature treatments) cryothérapie *f*

crypt (small concave area of organ) crypte *f*

crystalline lens (in eye) cristallin *m*

crunch, to croquer

cubic millimetre (mm^3) millimètre cube (abbrev. to mm3)

cupping glass (applied to skin for counterirritation treatment) ventouse *f*

curare (an anaesthetic) curare *m*

curable guérissable *adj*

cure guérison *f*

cure, to guérir *v*

curettage curetage *m*

curette curette *f*

curvature of the spine; scoliosis déviation *f* de la colonne; scoliose *f*

to the left scoliose *f* sinistroconvexe

to the right scoliose *f* dextroconvexe

Cushing's syndrome (overproduction of gluocortoids) syndrome *m* de Cushing

cut coupe *f*; plaie *f*

cut, accidental solution *f* de continuité

cut/sore, small bobo *m* (used when speaking to young children)

cyanosis, congenital (bluish skin due to oxygen deficiency) cyanose *f* ; maladie *f* bleue

cyanosis, person affected by; body area affected by cyanosé(e) *m/f*

cyst kyste *m*

cyst, fatty lipome *m*; loupe *f*

cyst, internal lésion *f* kystique

cystic kystique *adj*

cystic lesion lésion *f* kystique

cystic fibrosis (hereditary disease usually leading to respiratory infection) fibrose *f* kystique

cystitis (bladder inflammation) cystite *f*

cystoscopy (internal examination of bladder using a fibrescope) cystoscopie *f*

cytology (study of cells) cytologie *f*

cytobacteriological examination (for cells and microbes in urine) examen *m* cytobactériologique des urines *f* (ECBU)

damage, to léser *v*

dandruff pellicules *fpl*

dandruff lotion lotion *f* contre les pellicules

dark glasses lunettes *f* noires

deadly nightshade belladonne *f*

deaf sourd(e) *adj*

deaf-aid appareil *m* acoustique; audiophone *m*

deaf-and-dumbness surdimutité *f*

deafness surdité *f*

deafness, partial subcophose *m*

death mort *f*

death by drowning mort *f* par noyade *f*

decayed carié(ée) *adj*

decease décès *m*

deceased person défunt *m*, défunte *f*

decibel décibel *m*

decongestant décongestif *m*

decongestant décongestif -ive *adj*

defecation défécation *f*; déjection *f*

deficiency disease (gen. term) maladie *f* de/par carence *f*

deformation déformation *f*

defibrillator (electrical apparatus to revive heart) défibrillateur *m*

defibrillation défibrillation *f*

deformity déformation *f*

degenerate dégénéré(e) *m/f*

degeneration dégénération *f*

deglutition (swallowing) déglutition *f*

degree degré *m*

degree Baumé (density scale for liquids) degré *m* Baumé

dehydrated déshydraté(e) *adj*

dehydration déshydratation *f*

delirious, to be délirer *v*

delirium tremens (psychosis caused by chronic alcoholism) delirium tremens *m*

deliver, to (child) accoucher *v*
delivery (at childbirth) dégagement *m*
delivery, induced accouchement *m* provoqué
delivery accouchement *m*
deltoid (shoulder muscle) deltoïde *m*
delusion fantasme *m*
demented person dément(e) *m/f*
dementia démence *f*
dementia, senile démence *f* sénile
demineralisation (abnormal calcium loss in bones) déminéralisation *f*
demulcent émollient *m*
dengue fever (tropical disease causing acute joint pains) dengue *f*
dental dentaire *adj*
dental amalgam amalgame *m* dentaire
dental care soins *mpl* dentaires
dental floss fil *m* dentaire
dental plaque plaque *f* dentaire
dental plate dentier *m*
dental pulp (physiological tissue inside tooth) pulpe *f* dentaire
dental surgery work chirurgie *f* dentaire
dental technician mécanicien *m* –ne *f* dentiste
dental technique art *m* dentaire
dental treatment traitement *m* dentaire
dentine (bony substance forming the tooth) dentine *f*
dentist dentiste *m/f*
dentistry dentisterie *f*; odontologie *f*
dentition formule *f* dentaire; dentition *f*
denture dentier *m*
dependent dépendant(e) *m/f* and *adj*
depilatory (agent that removes unwanted hair) dépilatoire *m*
deposit dépôt *m*
depressed neurasthénique *adj*
depressed person neurasthénique *m* and *f*
depression dépression *f*; neurasthénie *f*

depression, disguised (no usual symptoms) dépression *f* masquée

depression, moderate/slight dépression *f* modérée/légère

depression, neurotic (unusually serious) dépression *f* névrotique

depression, person affected by dépressif *m* -ive *f* *adj*

depression following physical or emotional shock dépression *f* réactionnelle

depression (with loss of willpower) aboulie *f*

depressive dépressif *m* -ive *f* *adj*

dermatitis (skin inflammation) dermatite *f*

dermatological soap savon *m* dermatologique

dermatologist (skin specialist) dermatologiste *m*

dermatology (study/practice of) dermatologie *f*

dermatosis (skin disease) dermatose *f*

desensitisation (to allergies) désensibilisation *f*

destruction (of cells) cytolyse *f*

detached, to become abnormally se décoller *v*

detachment (of organism, etc.), abnormal décollement *m*

detect, to (illness, disease) dépister *v*

deteriorate, to altérer *v*

deterioration dégénerescence *f*

detoxification désintoxication *f*

detoxify, to désintoxiquer *v*

develop, to (illness) évoluer *v*

development (growth of child, adolescent) croissance *f*

development (illness) croissance *f*; évolution *f*

development (of medicines) mise *f* au point

devil's claw (plant) griffe *f* du diable

dextrose dextrose *f*

diabetes diabète *m*

diabetes, medical practice/study of diabétologie *f*

diabetes mellitus (sweet diabetes) diabète *m* sucré

diabetes mellitus requiring daily insulin injections insulinodépendant(e) *adj*

diabetes specialist diabétologue *m/f*

diabetes sufferer diabètique *m/f*
diabetes, to have être diabétique; avoir du diabète
diabetic diabétique *adj.*
diabetic coma coma *m* diabétique
diagnose, to diagnostiquer *v*
diagnostic diagnostique *adj.*
diagnostic computer ordinateur *m* de diagnostic
diagnostic investigations (blood tests, observation) recherche *f* diagnostique
diagnostic test/observations recherche *f* diagnostique
dialyser dialyseur *m*
dialysis épuration *f* extrarénale; dialyse *f*
dialysis machine rein *m* artificiel
dialysis unit unité *f* de dialyse
diaphragm (muscle area separating chest from stomach) coupole *f* diaphragmatique
diarrhoea diarrhée *f*
diastole (intervals between heart contractions when the chambers fill with blood) diastole *f* (see also **systole**)
diastolic blood pressure tension artérielle *f* diastolique
die, to décéder; mourir; trouver *v* la mort
diet diète *f*; régime *m*
diet (of food/drink) diètique; light *adj.*
diet, to be on a suivre *v* un régime
dietician diéticien *m* -ne *f*
diffuse diffus(e) *adj*
digest, to digérer *v*
digestibility digestibilité *f*
digestion digestion *f*; transit *m* intestinal
digestive digestif -ive *adj.*
digestive disorder trouble *m* digestif
digestive glands glandes *fpl* digestives
digestive organs organes *mpl* digestifs
digestive system appareil *m* digestif; système *m* digestif
digestive tract bacteria entérobactérie *f*
digital digital(e) (*pl* -aux) *adj*
digitalin (pharmaceutical properties of foxglove used

for certain heart condition) digitaline *f*
dilatation dilatation *f*
dilatation of blood vessels, drug causing; minoxidil minoxidil *m*
dilate, to dilater *v*
dilator (muscle) dilatateur *m*
dimunition décroissance *f*
dimunition of red corpuscles déglobulisation *f*
dip-test (for substance in blood or urine) bandelette *f*
diphtheria diphtérie *f*
directions for use (medicines) mode d'emploi *m*; posologie *f*
disability handicap *m*
disabled handicapé(e) *m/f*; invalide *adj*
disabled person handicapé(e) *m/f*; invalide *m* and *f*
disabled person, industrially invalide *m* and *f* du travail
disabled person, severely grand/e *m/f* invalide civil
disc disque *m*
disc, slipped hernie *f* discale
discharge, to (from the body) évacuer *v*; laisser écouler *v*
discharge, to (in-patient) renvoyer *v*
discharge oneself, to (from hospital) signer *v* sa décharge
disease (see also illness and illnesses list) affection *f*; maladie *f*
disease, chronic maladie *f* chronique
disease, contagious maladie *f* contagieuse
disease, fatal maladie *f* mortelle
disease transmissible to humans from animals; zoonosis zoonose *f*
disinfect, to désinfecter *v*
disinfectant pommade *f* anti-infection *f*; produit *m* désinfectant
disinfection désinfection *f*
disinfection and cleaning of wound détersion *f*
dislocate, to déboîter; démettre; disloquer; luxer
dislocate one's wrist/shoulder etc., to se démettre le poignet *m*/ l'épaule *f* etc.
dislocated démis(e) *adj.*
dislocation dislocation *f*; luxation *f*

disorder(s) trouble(s) *m*
disposable nappy couche-culottte *f*; couche *f* jetable
disposable razor rasoir *m* jetable
distended spleen dilatation *f* de la rate
diverticulitis (inflammation of a diverticulum) diverticulite *f*
diverticulum (abnormal tube in alimentary tract) diverticule *m*
divination power, using pendulum over body radiesthésie *f*
diving goggles lunettes *fpl* de plongée
diuretic diurétique *m*
diuretic diurétique *adj.*
diuretic medicine/drug spironolactone *f*
divisible or scored (pill, tablet) sécable *adj*
dizziness vertige *m*
dizzy spell étourdissement *m*
dizzy spell, to have a avoir *v* un éblouissement *m*
doctor docteur; Dr. *m* (form of address) ; médecin *m* (referring to a doctor)
doctor consulted by another doctor (médecin) consultant *m*
doctor, army (medical officer) médecin *m* militaire
doctor, company (for employees) médecin *m* du travail
doctor, duty médecin *m* de garde
doctor, school médecin *m* scolaire
doctor's instructions/ recommendations prescription *f*
doctor's report observation *f* médicale
doctor's written report of what a patient says allégation *f*
dome of the skull calotte *f* crânienne; voûte *f* crânienne
donation (of organs) don *m* d'organes
donor donneur *m* -euse *f*
dopamine (compound in nervous tissue) dopamine *f*
dorsal dorsal(e) (*pl* -aux) *adj*

dorsal vertebrae vertèbres *fpl* cervicales

dosage dosage *m*

dose dose *f*

Down's syndrome syndrome *m* de Down

Down's syndrome person trisomique *m/f*

drain, to drainer

drainage drainage *m*

drainage tube drain *m*

drained, to feel avoir *v* un coup de pompe

draw-sheet alaise *f*, alèze *f*

draw-sheet, single-use alaise/alèze *f* jetable

dream rêve *m*

dress, to (wound) mettre *v* un pansement; panser

dressing pansement *m*

to put a clean dressing on refaire *v* un pansement

drink, to boire; s'hydrater (take in moisture)

drip; perfusion perfusion *f*

drip, to put someone on a alimenter *v* au goutte-au-goutte

drip, to be put on a se mettre *v* sous perfusion

drip, hypertonic (containing extremely concentrated liquid) perfusion *f* hypertonique

drip (feed) (système) goutte-à-goutte *m*

drip feeding drip *m* feeding; perfusion *f*

drip transfusion drip *m* transfusion

dripping nose goutte *f* au nez

drop (of liquid) goutte *f*

dropper (pipette) compte-gouttes *m*

dropsy anasarque *f* hydropisie; œdème *m*

drowning noyade *f*

drowsiness somnolence *f*

drug (medicine) médicament *m*

drug (narcotic) narcotique *m*; stupéfiant *m*

drug drogue *f*

drug, hard/soft drogue *f* dure/douce

drug addict drogué(e) *m/f*; intoxiqué(e) *m/f*; toxicomane *m/f*

drug addicted toxicomane *adj*

drug addiction toxicomanie *f*

drug addiction, treatment for cure *f* de désintoxication
drug dependency pharmacodépendance *f*
drug substitute (for drug addicts) sevrage *m* pharmacologique
dry dressing pansement *m* sec
dry out, to (from alcoholism) désintoxiquer
duct canal *m*; conduit *m*; vaisseau *m*; voie *f*
dumbness mutité *f*
dummy sucette *f*; tétine *f*
duodenal duodénal(e) *adj*
duodenal ulcer ulcère *f* duodénale; ulcère *m* du duodénum
duodenum duodénum *m*
duodenum, inflammation of duodénite *f*
dura mater (outermost membrane around the brain and spinal cord) dure-mère *f*
dwarfism nanisme *m*
dysentery dysenterie *f*
dysfunction dysfonctionnement *m*
dyslexia dyslexie *f*
dyslexic dyslexique *adj*
dysmenorrhea (painful or difficult menstruation) dysménorrhée *f*
dyspepsia dyspepsie *f*
dysphasia (speech disorder) dysphasie *f*
dysplasia (abnormal tissue growth) dysplasie *f*
dyspnoea (laboured breathing) dyspnée *f*
dystrophy dystrophie *f*
dysuria (painful/difficult urination) dysurie *f*

ear oreille *f*
ear (concerning) auriculaire *adj*
ear, inner oreille *f* interne
ear, outer oreille *f* externe
ear, outer part of pavillon *m* de l'oreille
earache mal *m* aux oreilles
eardrum tympan *m*
eardrum injury (explosions, altitude, scuba diving) barotraumisme *m*
ear drops gouttes *f* pour les oreilles
ear inflammation/infection, of outer/inner ear; otitis otite *f* (externe/interne)

ear lobe lobe *m* de l'oreille

ear, nose and throat department département *m*/service *m* d'oto-rhino-laryngolie

ear, nose and throat medicine (specialty) médecine *f* oto-rhino-laryngologie *f*

ear, nose and throat specialist oto-rhino-laryngologiste *m and f*

ear passage to eardrum méat *m* auditif

ear plug (for keeping out water) bouchon *m* d'oreille (pour l'eau)

ear plug (for keeping out noise) boule *f* Quies ® (pour bruit)

ear tumour (following repeated infection) cholestéatome *m*

early (diagnosis) précoce *adj*

early signs/stages (of illness) ébauche *f*

earwax cérumen *m*

ease (relieve), to soulager *v*

Ebola virus disease maladie *f* à virus *m* Ebola

echocardiography (ultrasound heart scan) échocardiographie *f*

echography (ultrasound scanning) échographie *f*

eclampsia; convulsions éclampsie *f*

ectopic preganancy (fœtus outside womb) grossesse *f* extra-utérine

eczema eczéma *m*

eczema (affecting babies) eczéma *m* atopique

eczema following (allergic) contact eczéma *m* de contact

eczetamous disease affecting hands and feet dys(h)idrose *f*

edge (of a cut/incision/wound) berge *f*; lèvres *f* d'une incision/plaie

edgy nerfs *mpl* à vif (idiom)

edible comestible *adj*

effusion (abnormal presence of liquid) épanchement *m*

elastic band bande *f* élastique

elastic support bandage bande *f* de tissu élastique

elasticity compliance *f*

elbow coude *m*

elbow bone; olecranon olécrâne *m*

elbow joint; epicondyle épicondyle *m*

elderly, the personnes *fpl* âgées

elderly person who is no longer physically independent personne *f* âgée dépendante

electric blanket couverture *f* chauffante

electric lounging armchair with help-you-up function fauteuil *m* électrique avec fonction releveur

electric shock choc *m* électrique; commotion *f* électrique; décharge *f* électrique

electrocardiogram (record of heart's electrical activity) électrocardiogramme *m* (ECG)

electrocardiograph (instrument which records heart's electrical activity) électrocardiographe *m*

electroencephalogram (record's brain electrical activity) électroencéphalogramme *m* (EEG)

electroencephalograph (examination of brain's electrical activity) électroencéphalographe *m*

electronic monitoring surveillance *f* électronique

electrocution électrocution *f*

electrolytes electrolytes *f*

electrotherapy électrothérapie *f*

eliminate, to éliminer *v*

elimination élimination *f*

elongation of large intestine (not an illness) dolichocôlon *m*

embolism (blood clot or air bubble blockage) embolie *f*

embolism, air embolie *f* gazeuse

embolism, arterial embolie *f* artérielle

embolism, cerebral embolie *f* cérébrale

embolism, pulmonary embolie *f* pulmonaire

embrocation embrocation *f*

embryo embryon *m*

embryology embryologie *f*

embryonic embryonnaire *adj*

embryonic condition à l'état *m* d'embryon

emergency urgence *f*
emetic (medicine which causes vomiting) émétique *m*
emphysema (lung condition causing breathlessness) emphysème *m*
empirical remedy remède *m* empirique
empty stomach, on an (required before many blood tests) à jeun
emulsion (medicinal) émulsion *f*
enamel (tooth) émail *m*
encephalitis (inflammation of the brain) encéphalite *f*
encephalogram (brain X-ray) encéphalogramme *m*
encephalon (brain and top of spinal cord) encéphale *f*
endemic endémique *adj*
endocardium (inner wall of the heart) endocarde *m*
endocardium, inflammation of endocardite *f*
endocrine system (glands) système *m* endocrinien
endocrine glands (ovaries, testicles, thyroid) glandes *fpl* endocrines
endocrine system système *m* endocrinien
endocrinology endocrinologie *f*
endogenous (originating from body interior) endogène *adj*
endometrium (membrane lining the uterus) endomètre *m*
endometriosis (inflammation of the uterus lining) endométriose *f*
endorphine (morphine-like substance produced by brain) endorphine *f*
endoscope (instrument for internal examinations) endoscope *m*
endoscopy examination endoscopie *f*
enema (rectum injection) lavement *m*
enema (fluid used) lavement *m*
enema, barium (pre X-rays: coloscopy more usual) lavement *m* barite
engorge, to engorger *v*
engorgement engorgement *m*
enteritis (small intestine inflammation) entérite *f*

enterobacteria (digestive tract bacteria) entérobactérie *f*

enterobiasis (pinworm/threadworm illness) oxurose *f*

enterocolitis (inflammation of large and small intestines) entérocolite *f*

enterovirus (intestinal virus which can spread elsewhere) entérovirus *m*

enzyme (biological substance aiding/allowing chemical reaction) enzyme *m/f*

epicondyle (elbow joint) épicondyle *m*

epidemic épidémie *f*

epidemic threshold seuil *m* épidémique

epidermis épiderme *m*

epidural péridurale *f*

epidural (relating to the outermost membrane around brain and spinal cord) péridural(e) (*pl* -aux) *adj*

epidural anaesthesia (into lower area of spinal cord) anesthésie *f* péridurale

epidymis (duct behind testicles) épididyme *m*

epidymis inflammation épididymite *f*

epiglottis épiglotte *f*

epilation (hair removal) épilation *f*

epilepsy épilepsie *f*

epilepsy, severe comitialité *f*, épilespsie *f* généralisée

epileptic fit crise *f* d'épilepsie

epileptic fits, successive état *m* de mal épileptique

episiotomy (surgical cut into vagina to aid childbirth) épisiotomie *f*

epithelial tissue (body and digestive tract tissue) tissu *m* épithélial

epithelioma (malignant tumour of epithelial tissue) épithélioma *m*

epithelium (body surface, digestive tract and other cavity tissue) epithelium *m*

ergonomic ergonomique *adj*

ergonomic seat cover for back support sursiège *m* soutien de dos

erosion of joints érosion *f*; écorchure *f*

eruption (of teeth growing through the gums) éruption *f*
eruption of blisters; vesicatory vésicatoire *m*
erysipelas (reddish skin infection) érysipèle *m*
erythema (abnormal redness of the skin) érythème *m*
Escherichia coli (E. coli) Escherichia coli *m*
essential oil (used in medicines) huile *f* essentielle
established (through tests, of illness) avéré(e) *adj*
ethics, medical déontologie *f* médicale
ethmoid bone (above nose and behind forehead) ethmoïde *m*
etiology/aetiology (study of disease causes) étiologie *f*
euthanasia euthanasie *f*
evacuate, to (from body) évacuer *v*
evacuation déjection *f*
evacuation (draining of liquid) évacuation *f*
evacuation (vomiting) rejet *m*
evening (of symptoms, etc.) vespéral(e) (*pl* -aux) *adj*
evolution évolution *f*
evolve, to (of illness) évoluer *v*
exacerbation exacerbation *f*
examine, to examiner *v*
examination investigation *f*
examination, complementary examen *m* complémentaire
examination, detailed exploration *f*
examination of the exterior of the cervix examen *m* exocervical
examination room salle *f* d'examens *m*
excite, to exciter *v*
exceed, to dépasser *v*
excrement déjections *fpl*
excretion excrétion *f*
exercise bike vélo *m* d'appartement ; vélo *m* d'intérieur
exhausted, to feel avoir *v* un coup de pompe
exhausted state, (utterly) (grand) état *m* d'épuisement
exhaustion coup *m* de pompe (informal); épuisement *m*
exophthalmia (abnormally globular eyes) exophtalmie *f*

expectorant expectorant *m* and *adj*

exploration (detailed examination) exploration *f*

exploratory explorateur -rice; exploratoire *adj*

exploratory operation intervention *f* exploratrice

extensor muscle extenseur *m*

external; exterior externe *adj*

external use (only) (à) usage *m* externe

extract, to arracher *v*; extraire *v*

extraction extraction *f*

extrasystole (irregular heartbeat) extrasystole *f* auriculaire

eye oeil *m* (*pl* yeux)

eye, black oeil *m* poché; oeil au beurre noir

black/dark rings under eyes yeux *m* battus

eyes, blood-shot yeux *m* injectés de sang

eyes, dryness of sécheresse *f* oculaire

eye astigmatism astigmatisme *m*

eye drops gouttes *f* pour les yeux

eye exercises gymnastique *f* oculaire

eye inflammation; ophthalmia ophtalmie *f*

eye socket orbite *f*

eye solution solution *f* oculaire

eye specialist ophtalmologiste *m/f*; ophtalmologue *m/f*; oculiste *m/f*

eye surgery chirurgerie *f* ophtalmique

eye wash bain *m* d'oeil; bain *m* oculaire

eyeball globe *m* oculaire

eyeball membrane choroïde *f*

eyebath œillère *f*

eyebrow sourcil *m*

eyecup œillère *f*

eyelash cil *m*

eyelid paupière *f*

eyelid, closed (stuck) occlusion *f* palpébrale

eyelids (concerning) palpébralé(e) (*pl* -aux) *adj*

eyelid, lower/upper paupière *f* inférieure/supérieure

eyelid abscess chalazion *f*

eyelid inflammation; blepharitis blépharite *f*

eyelid membrane conjonctive *f*

eyesight vision *f*
eyesight test test *m* d'acuité *f* visuelle
eyesight trouble trouble *m* de la vision

face visage *m*; face *f*
face cream crème *f* pour le visage
face-lift (plastic or cosmetic surgery) lifting *m*
facial facial(e) *adj*
facial nerve nerf *m* facial
facial paralysis paralysie *f* faciale
facial surgery chururgie *f* faciale
factor (as in protection factors for sun lotion) facteur *m*
faeces matières *f* fécales
faeces, dark (bloody) méléna/melaena *m*
faint, to s'évanouir *v*; tomber *v* en syncope; tomber *v* dans les pommes *f* (informal)
fainting perte *f* de connaissance
fainting fit/spell évanouissement *m*; syncope *f*
faintness/sickness (feeling of) défaillance *f*; malaise *m*
fall, to tomber *v*
Fallopian tube trompe *f* de Fallope
Fallopian tube, removal of annexectomie *f*
Fallot's congenital heart-valve malformation tétralogie *f* de Fallot
family planning planification *f* familiale; planning *m* familial
Fanconi disease (congenital illness causing poor reproduction of red corpuscles) maladie *f* de Fanconi
fantasy fantasme *m*
fast, to jeûner *v*
fasting jeûne *m*
fatal disease/illness maladie *f* mortelle
fatigue fatigue *f*
fat-soluble liposoluble *adj*
fattiness in female buttocks; steatopygy stéatopygie *f*
fatty acid/oils/wax/steroid; lipid lipide *m*
fatty cyst lipome *m*; loupe *f*

fatty cysts, presence of lipomatose *f*

fatty tissue tissu *m* adipeux

fatty tissue build-up infiltration *f* graisseuse

features faciès *m*

febrifuge (treatment to prevent/reduce fever) fébrifuge *m* and *adj*; antipyrétique *m* and *adj*

feeble faible *adj*

feebleness asthénie *f*

feed up, to suralimenter *v*

feeding tube sonde *f* d'alimentation

feeding up therapy suralimentation *f*

feel, to sentir *v*

feel unwell, to ne pas se sentir *v* bien

femoral quadriceps (four-headed thigh muscle) quadriceps *m* (fémoral)

femur fémur *m*

femur, broken neck of col *m* du fémur caissé

fennel (plant) fenouil *m*

fermentation culture ferment *m* lactique

fertility fécondité *f*; fertilité *f*

fertility drug médicament *m* contre la stérilité

fertilisation fécondation *f*

festering ulcéreux -euse *adj*

fever fièvre *f*

fever, absence of apyrexie *f*

fever (recurring every four days) fièvre *f* quartane

fever attack accès *m* de fièvre

feverish fièvreux -euse *adj*

feverish convulsions convulsions *fpl* fébriles

feverish person fébrile *m/f*

fibrescope (optic fibres instrument enabling internal examination) fibroscope *f*

fibrescope examination fibroscopie *f*

fibrillation (quivering movement, especially of heart muscle) fibrillation *f*

fibrillation, auricular fibrillation *f* auriculaire (FA)

fibrillation, ventricular fibrillation *f* ventriculaire (FV)

fibroid in the uterus fibrome *m* de l'utérus

fibrositis aponévrite *f*

fibrous swelling on scar chéloïde *f*

fibula (lower and outer leg bone) péroné *m*

fill, to (teeth) obturer *v*

fill a tooth provisionally, to panser *v*

filling (in tooth) plombage *m*

filling, to lose a perdre un plombage *m*

finger doigt *m*

finger, index index *m*

finger, little auriculaire *m*

finger, middle majeur *m*

finger, third annulaire *m*

finger bone; phalanx phalange *f*

fingernail ongle *m* de la main

fingerprint empreinte *f* digitale

fingerstall (cover to protect a finger) doigtier *m*

fireman pompier *m*; sapeurs-pompiers *m*

first aid premiers *m* soins

first-aid box trousse *f* d'urgence

first-aid kit trousse *f* de premier secours; trousse *f* de premiers soins; trousse *f* à pharmacie

first-aid manual manuel *m* de premiers soins

first-aid post poste *m* de secours

first-degree burn brûlure *f* du premier degré

fissure sillon *m*

fissure of the brain, longitudinal scissure *f* interhémisphérique

fist poignet *m*

fistula (abnormal passage between organs) fistule *f*

fit attaque *f*

fit, to (an appliance or artificial limb) poser *v*

fit, to throw a piquer *v* une crise

fitful (of sleep) troublé; agité *adj*

fitful (esp. of breathing, pulse) irrégulier *m* -ère *f adj*

fitness forme *f* physique

flaking skin condition; pityriasis pityriasis *m*

flask flacon *m*

flat plat -e *adj*

flat-footed aux pieds *m* plats

flatulence flatulence *f*

flatus flatuosité *f*

flavour parfum *m*

flavouring (for medicines) excipient *m*
flex, to fléchir *v*
flexor muscle fléchisseur *m*
flu grippe *f*
flu, bad attack of mauvaise grippe *f*
flu vaccine vaccin *m* de grippe
fluke (parasitic flatworm) distome *m*; douve *f*
fluoridation (of water, helping to preserve teeth) fluoration *f*
fluoride toothpaste dentifrice *m* fluoré
fluorine fluor *m*
fluoride fluorure *m*
flush flush *m*
focussing function (of eyes); accommodation accommodation *f*
foetus foetus *m*
foetus communication through sensory stimulation haptonomie *f*
follicle (small cavity, sac or gland) follicule *m*
follicle, inflammation of folliculite *f*
follow treatment, to suivre *v* une thérapie
fontanelle (boneless part of a baby's head) fontanelle *f*
food hygiene hygiène *f* alimentaire
food poisoning intoxication *f* alimentaire; toxi-infection *f* alimentaire
food-poisoning infection; listeriosis listériose *f*
food rich/poor in vitamins alimentation *f* riche/pauvre en vitamines
food supplement complément *m* alimentaire
food wedged between teeth bourrage *f* alimentaire
foods for dieting aliments *m* de régime
foot pied *m*
foot bone métatarse *m*
foot/hand pedalling exercise machine pédalier *m*
foot massager (appliance) appareil *m* de massage pour les pieds
forceps forceps *m*
forearm avant-bras *m*
forearm bone; ulna cubitus *m*

forefinger index *m*
forehead front *m*
forehead bone (frontal) os *m* frontal
foreign body corps *m* étranger
forensic medicine reports expertises *f* de médecine légale
forensic scientist expert *m* légiste
forensic surgeon médecin *m* légiste
foreskin prépuce *m*
foreskin, abnormal covering of (in young boy) adhérence *f* préputiale
fracture fracture *f*
fracture, clean fracture *f* en bois vert
fracture, closed fracture *f* fermée
fracture, Colles' arm (lower radius) fracture *f* de Pouteau-Colles
fracture, compound fracture *f* ouverte
fracture, simple fracture *f* fermée
fracture, to set/reduce réduire *v*
fracture, to fracturer *v*
fracture which can be reduced/set, of réductible *adj*
fracture which cannot be reduced/set, of irréductible *adj*
fracture due to excessive physical activity fracture *f* de fatigue
fracture of the skull fracture *f* du crâne
fractured arm/leg/rib bras *m* cassé/jambe *f* cassée/côte *f* cassée
fractured skull enfoncement *m* de la boîte crânienne
free radical (constant element/atom part of chemical compound) radical *m* libre
frostbite gelure *f*
frozen embryo embryon *m* congelé
fumigator fumigateur *m*
functional disorder désordre *m* fonctionnel; trouble *m* fonctionnel
functional failure of organ défaillance *f*
functioning fonctionnement *m*

funduscopy (examination of back of the eye) examen *m* du fond de l'oeil
fungal disease; mycosis mycose *f*
fungal disease affecting nails; onychomycosis onychomycose *f*
fungal diseases, medicine for treatment of antimycosique *f*
fungus champignon *m* (generic term); mycose *f* (med.)
fungi specialist mycologiste *m*
furuncle (boil) furoncle *m*

galenic (of medicine produced from animal or vegetable tissue) galénique *adj*
gall bladder vésicule *f* biliaire
gall bladder, inflammation of cholécystite *f*
gall bladder, surgical removal of; cholycystectomy cholécystectomie *f*
gall bladder, X-ray of cholécystographie *f*
gall stone calcul *m* biliaire
gamma rays rayons *m* gamma
ganglion (nerve cluster/nucleus) ganglion *m*
ganglion disorders adénopathie *f*
gangrene gangrène *f*
gargle gargarisme *m*
gargle, to se faire *v* un gargarisme
garlic ail *m*
gastrectomy (surgical removal of whole/part of stomach) gastrectomie *f*
gastric gastrique *adj*
gastric acidity acidité *f* gastrique
gastric flu grippe *f* gastro-intestinale
gastric ulcer ulcère *m* de l'estomac
gastritis (inflammation of stomach lining) gastrite *f*
gastro-enteritis (inflammation of stomach and intestines) gastroentérite *f*
gastric flu grippe *f* intestinale
gastroenteroligist (digestion specialist) gastroenterologue *m*
gastroenterology gastroentérologie *f*
gastroenterology department service *m* de gastroentérologie
gauze compress compresse *f* de gaze

gelatine capsule gélule *f*
gene therapy thérapie *f* génique
general anaesthesia anésthésie *f* générale
general surgery chirurgerie *f* générale
genetic code codage *m* génétique
genetic material matériel *m* génétique
generalise, to généraliser *v*
generalised (of infection) systématisé(e) *adj*
genetic génétique *adj*
genetic advice (for future parents using hereditary illnesses) conseil *m* génétique
genetic engineering génie *m* génétique; manipulations *f* génétiques
genetic figerprint empreinte *f* génétique
genetically modified organism (e.g. cereal grains) (GMO) organisme *m* génétiquement modifié (OGM)
genetics génétique *f*
genital blisters/warts vésicules *fpl* génitales
genital herpes herpes *m* génital
genital organs organes (*mpl.*) génitaux
genitals sexe *m*
genome génome *m*
genotype (genetic constitution of a person) génotype *m*
gentian (gentian violet dye is used as antiseptic) gentiane *f*
geriatric gériatrique *adj*
geriatric ward service *m* gériatrique
geriatrics gériatrie *f*
germ germe *m*; microbe *m*
German camomile camomille *f* allemande
German measles rubéole *f*
German measles vaccine vaccin *m* contre la rubéole
gerontology gérontologie *f*
gestation gestation *f*
giddiness vertige *m*
giddiness, fit of étourdissement *m*
gingival gingival(e) *adj*
gingivitis gingivite *f*
ginseng (root powder) ginseng *m*
gland glande *f*

glanders (contagious disease affecting jaws and nostrils, transmitted by horses) morve *f*
glandular glandulaire *adj*
glandular fever fièvre *f* ganglionnaire/glandulaire; mononucléose *f* infectieuse
glasses (eyesight) lunettes *f*
Glauber's salt (sodium sulphate) sel *m* de Glauber
glaucoma (diminishing eyesight) glaucome *m*
glottis (upper end of windpipe) glotte *f*
glucose glucose *m*
glucoses (normal and stable amounts of different types in the blood) équilibre *m* glycémique
glucose (tolerance) test épreuve *f* de tolérance *f* au glucose; épreuve *f* d'hyperglycémie *f* provoquée
gluteal (buttock) muscles muscles *m* fessiers
gluten (protein present in cereal grains) gluten *m*
glycaemia (glucose level in blood) glycémie *f*
glycerine glycerol (used as laxative) glycerine *f* glycérol
glycerol used in small doses as laxative polyéthylène *m* glycol (PEG)
goitre (neck swelling) goitre *m*
gonad (ovary or testicle) gonade *f*
gonadotropin (substance stimulating gonads to produce sperm/egg) gonadotrophine *f*
gonalgy (knee pain) gonalgie *f*
gonorrhoea blennoragie *f*; gonorrhée *f*
gout goutte *f*
govt. health assurance medical officer médecin *m* conseil
GP médecin *m* généraliste
GP linked to health scheme (after changes were announced in 1998) médecin *m* référent
graft greffe *f*
graft, to greffer *v*
graft using healthy tissue from patient's own body autogreffe *f*

gravel (stones in urinary tract) gravelle *f*
gravel (crystals formed in urinary tract) lithiase *f* urinaire
graze éraflure *f*
greater plantain (plant, used as mild laxative) plantain *m* majeur
grinding (of teeth) mâchonnement *m*
gripe water calmant *m* pour coliques infantiles
gripes (violent stomach pains) coliques *f*; tranchées *f*
gripping (ability) préhension *f*
groin aine *f*
groin or neck pulses pouls *mpl* centraux
groove (in bone) gouttière *f*
group therapy thérapie *f* de groupe
growing pains (child development) épiphysite *f*
growth, benign adénome *m*
growth, benign (often on a breast) adénofibrome *m*
growth (fleshy) on a healing cut granulome *m*
growth (small and harmless); papilloma papillome *m*
growth (of adolescent, child) croissance *f*
grumbling appendicitis appendicite *f* chronique
gullet; oesophagus œsophage *m*
gullet, abnormal closing up of achalasie *f*
gullet and stomach surgery (partial removal); oesogastrectomy oesogastrectomie *f*
gullet inflammation due to stomach acids oesophagite *f* peptique
gum (teeth) gencive *f*
gum ointment pâte *f* gingivale
gumboil abcès *m* à la gencive; fluxion *f* dentaire
gumma (internal tissue swelling) gomme *f*
gustative gustatif -ive *adj*
gymnastics gymnastique *f*
gynaecologist gynécologue *m/f*
gynaecology gynécologie *f*
gynaecology unit unité *f* gynécologique

haematological hématologique *adj*
haematologist (blood specialist) hématologue *m/f*
haematology (study of blood) hématologie *f*
haematoma poche *f* de sang
haemodialysis (kidney dialysis) hémodialyse *f*
haemoglobin (red oxygen-carrying protein in blood) hémoglobine *f*
haemolysis (loss of haemoglobin) hémolyse *f*
haemolysis, pathological (abnormal elimination of red corpuscles) hémolyse *f* pathologique
haemolysis, physiological (natural elimination of red corpuscles) hémolyse *f* physiologique
haemophilia (hereditary condition with failure of normal blood coagulation) hémophilie *f*
haemophiliac person hémophile *m/f*
haemophilic hémophile *adj*
haemorrhage hémorragie *f*
haemorrhage, external hémorragie *f* externe
haemorrhage, internal hémorragie *f* interne
haemorrhagic hémorragique *adj*
haemorrhoidal hémorroïdal(e) *adj*
haemorrhoids (piles) hémorroïdes *fpl*
haemorrhagic fever fièvre *f* hémorragique
haemostasis (stopping of haemorrhage) hémostase *f*
hair (body) poil *m*
hair (head) cheveux *mpl*
hair, fibrous proteins in; keratin kératine *f*
hair bulb bulbe *m* pileux
hair care soins *m* des cheveux
hair conditioner après-shampoing *m*; conditionneur *m*
hair cream pommade *f*
hair graft implant *m* capillaire
hair loss (temporary, partial or complete hair loss); alopecia alopécie *f*
hair, loss of chute *f* des cheveux *mp.*
hair loss, to cause dépiler *v*

hair care lotion lotion *f* capillaire

hair removal; epilation épilation *f*

hairline (of fracture) a minima *adj*

hair root cavity/gland follicule *m* pileux

hairy poilu(e) *adj*

hairy (plentiful body hair) système *m* pileux très développé

halitosis (bad breath) halitose *f*; mauvaise haleine *f*

hallucinated person; lunatic halluciné(e) *m/f*

hallucination hallucination *f*

hallucination, auditory (esp. voices) hallucination *f* auditive

hallucinations of seeing animals (associated with drug/drink addiction); zoopsy zoopsie *f*

hallucinatory delirium délire *m* hallucinatoire

hallucinogenic hallucinogène *adj*

ham (of leg) jarret *m*

hand main *f*

hand bone; metacarpus métacarpe *m*

hand cream crème *f* pour les mains

handicap handicap *m*

handicapped handicappé(e) *adj*

handicapped (physically) person déficient *m* -e *f* moteur

handicapped, to be permanently; handicapped for life rester handicapé(e) *m/f* à vie

hangover gueule *f* de bois

hard of hearing (person) malentendant(e) *adj*

hard palate voûte *f* du palais

harelip bec-de-lièvre *m*

hawthorn aubépine *f*

hay fever coryza *m* spasmodique des foins; rhume *m* des foins

head tête *f*

head (concerning the) céphalique *adj*

head, back of occiput *m*

headache; cephalagia céphaléé *f*; mal *m* de tête

headache, to have a avoir *v* mal à la tête

headaches, violent bouts of (without explanation) algie *f* vasculaire de la face

head cold coryza *m*; rhume *m* de cerveau

heal, to (of scar) cicatriser *v*; **(of illness)** guérir *v*

healing (of scar) cicatrisant(e) **(of illness)** guérison *adj*

healing product cicatrisant *m*

health santé *f*

health, in good/bad en bonne/ mauvaise santé *f*

health sanitaire *adj*

health care protection *f* contre les maladies

health/medical care/ treatment soins *m* médicaux

health care for mothers and young children protection *f* maternelle et infantile

health check up examen *m* de santé; bilan *m* de santé

health-food product produit *m* diétique

health insurance assurance *f* maladie

health record carnet *m* de santé; dossier *m* médical

healthier life, for a hygiène *f* de vie; pour une meilleure vie *f*

'healthy mind, healthy body' 'bien dans sa tête, bien dans son corps'

hearing ouïe *f*; audition *f*

hearing, to have a sharp sense of avoir l'ouië fine

hearing aid appareil *m* acoustique/auditif; audiophone *m*; prothèse *f* acoustique/ auditive

hearing decline (normal) with age presbyacousie *f*

hearing decline (premature) presbyacousie *f* précoce

hearing evaluation; acoumetry acoumétrie *f*

hearing one's own voice in the head, uncomfortable impression of autophonie *f*

heart coeur *m*

heart, weak cœur *m* fatigué

heart and blood circulation (study/treatment); cardiology cardiologie *f*

heart and blood circulation specialist; cardiologist cardiologue *m*

heart and blood-vessel conditions (medical

specialty) cardiologie *f*, affections *fpl* cardio-vasculaires

heart activity record over a 24 hour period Holter *m* rhythmique

heart area between auricles and ventricles jonction *f* atrio-ventriculaire /auriculo ventruculaire

heart artery disease coronaropathie *f*

heart attack crise *f* cardiaque; infarctus *m* du myocarde

heart attack, mild malaise *m* cardiaque

heart attack affecting the ventricular septum infarctus *m* septal

heart bypass operation pontage *m* cardiaque

heart disease cardiopathie *f*; maladie *f* du coeur

heart examination examen *m* cardiaque

heart failure défaillance *f* cardiaque

heart inflammation diseases; myocarditis myocardite *f*

heart irregularity intermittence *f*

heart kinetics (movement mechanics) cinétique *f* du coeur

heart muscle disease; cardiomyopathy cardiomyopathie *f*

heart murmur souffle *m* au coeur

heartrate rythme *m* du coeur

heartrate, abnormally fast; tachycardia tachycardie *f*

heartbeat, irregular extrasystole *f* auriculaire

heartbeats, irregular; arrhythmia arythmie *f*

heartbeat, irregular (with fast bursts); tachyarrythmia tachyarythmie *f*

heartbeat, medicine which restabilises antiarythmique *f*

heart membranes, inflammation of; carditis cardite *f*

heart-rate monitor moniteur *m* cardiaque

heart's auricle (concerning) auriculaire *adj*

heart surgeon cardiochirurgien(ne) *m/f*

heart surgery chirurgie *f* cardiaque
heart test ultrasound device doppler pulsé *m*
heart transplant greffe *f* du cœur; transplantation *f* cardiaque
heart valve valve *f* cardiaque
heart valve, artificial prothèse *f* valvulaire
heart valve (concerning) valvulaire *adj*
heart valve(s) deterioration atteinte *f* valvulaire
heart valve disease valvulopathie *f*
heart rate illness due to disorder in the heart's nerve centre tachycardia *f* jonctionnelle
heartbeat battement *m* de coeur
heartbeat noise, abnormal bruit *m* de galop
heartbeat, abnormal rubbing noise of frottement *m* péricardique
heartbeat, excessively fast (over 150 a minute) flutter *m*
heartbeat rate fréquence *f* cardiaque; rythme *m* cardiaque
heartbeat rate per minute battement *m* de coeur par minute (BPM)
heartburn aigreurs *m* d'estomac; brûlures *f* d'estomac
heat chaleur *f*
heat exhaustion épuisement *m* dû à la chaleur
heat treatment thermothérapie *f*
heatstroke coup *m* de chaleur
heel talon *m*
heel bone; calcaneum calcanéum *m*
height gauge/chart toise *f*
height and weight (concerning) staturo-pondéral(e) (*pl* -aux) *adj*
height-weight chart (for children) développement *m* staturo-pondéral
heliotherapy (sunlight treatment) héliothérapie *f*
hemiplegia (paralysis of one side of the body) hémiplégie *f*
hemiplegic (person paralysed down one side) hémiplégique *m/f*
hemiplegic (paralysed down one side) hémiplégique *adj*

heparin (anticoagulant in various organs and tissues) héparine f
hepatic (liver) colic colique *f* hépatique
hepatitis hépatite *f*
hepatitis A virus *m* de l'hépitate A (HAV)
hepatitis A vaccine vaccin *m* hépatite A
hepatitis B virus *m* de l'hépitate B (HAB)
hepatitis B vaccine vaccin hépatite B
hepatitis C virus *m* de l'hépitate C (HAC)
herbal medicine phytothérapie *f*
herbalist phytothérapeute *m and f*
hereditary héréditaire *adj*
hereditary disease maladie *f* héréditaire
hereditary bone growth reduction; achondroplasia achondroplasie *f*
heredity hérédité *f*
hermetically sealed plaster pansement *m* occlusif
hernia hernie *f*
hernia, hiatus (between chest and abdomen) hernie *f* hiatale
herpes herpès *m*
herpes zosta herpès *m* zosta
herpes zosta (concerning) zostérien(e) *adj*
hiccough; hiccup hoquet *m*
hiccough/hiccup, to hoqueter *v*
highly strung nerfs *m* fragiles
hip hanche *f*
hip area swelling with fever (temporary condition affecting children) rhume *m* de hanche; coxite transitoire *f*
hip bone os *m* iliaque
hip joint articulation *f* de la hanche; articulation *f* coxo-fémorale
hip-joint replacement operation arthroplastie *f* complète de la hanche *f*
hip replacement prothèse *f* de la hanche
hip replacement operation pose *f* d'une prothèse *f* de hanche
hippocampus (ridges at bottom of brain's lateral ventricles) hippocampe *m*

hirsutism (excessive hair growth) hirsutisme *m*
hissing sibilant(e) *adj*
hissing in ears sifflement *m*
histamine (body catalyst from allergies) histamine *f*
histology (study of tissues) histologie *f*
hives; urticaria urticaire *f*
Hodgkin's disease (cancerous) maladie *f* de Hodgkin
holistic (of treatment taking into account mental and social factors) holistique *adj.*
hollow/cavity (in the body) fosse *f*
hollow behind the knee creux *m* poplité
homeopathic homéopathique *adj*
homeopathic medicine/remedy médicament *m* homeopathique
homeopathy homeopathie *f*
homogeneous (aspect of healthy organs on X-rays, etc.) homogène *adj.*
hook-formed bone uncus *m*
hookworm ankylostome *m*
hookworm disease ankylostomiase *f*; ankylostomose *f*
hooping (metal wire repair technique to broken bone) cerclage *m* d'un os cassé
horizontal part of bone plateau *m*
hormone hormone *f*
hormone-producing gland disorder trouble *m* hormonal
hormone substitute (post-menopause) substitutif *m* hormonal
hormone treatment traitement *m* hormonal
horse chestnut preparation (not edible) marron *m* d'Inde
hospital hôpital *m* (*pl* -aux)
hospital ward/department service *m*
hot flush bouffée *f* de chaleur
house doctor interne/e *m/f* des hôpitaux
household soap savon *m* de Marseille
human body organisme *m*; corps *m* humain
human immunodeficiency virus (HIV) virus *m* de

l'immunodéficience *f* humaine (VIH)
human testing for new drugs essai *m* clinique
humerus (upper arm bone) humérus *m*
humour humeur *f*
hump gibbosité *f*
Huntington's chorea (with progressive dementia) chorée *f* de Huntington
hurt, to blesser *v*
hurt oneself, to se blesser *v*
hydration hydratation *f*
hydrocephalus (excessive fluid in the brain) hydrocéphalie *f*
hydrocortisone (steroid hormone for treating inflammations/rheumatism) hydrocortisone *f*
hydrogen peroxide eau *f* oxygénée
hydronephrosis (water-swollen kidney) hydronéphrose *f*
hydrotherapy hydrothérapie *f*
hygiene hygiène *f*
hygiene, body hygiène *f* corporelle
hygiene for good health hygiénisme *m*
hygiene at work hygiène du travail
hymen hymen *m*
hyperactive hyperactif -ive *adj.*
hyperglycaemia (glucose excess in bloodstream) hyperglycémie *f*
hyperhidrosis (excessive sweating) hyperhidrose *f*
hyperpathyroidisme (abnormal functioning of gland near the thyroid) hyperparathyroïdie *f*
hypertensive hypertensif -ive *adj.*
hypertension hypertension *f*
hyperthermia hyperthermia *f*
hypertonic (of high-tension muscles; of extremely concentrated medicine for injection) hypertonic *adj*
hypertonic drip perfusion *f* hypertonique
hypertrophy (organ/tissue enlargement due to increase in size of cells) hypertrophie *f*
hyperventilation (abnormally fast breathing rate) hyperventilation *f*

hypnosis hypnose *f*

hypnosis (using a magnet); hypnotism magnétisme *m*; mesmérisme *m*

hypnotherapy hypnothérapie *f*

hypnotic; sleep inducing (pill) hypnotique *m*

hypnotic hypnotique *adj*

hypoallergenic (of little/ reduced tendency to cause allergic reaction) hypoallergénique *adj*.

hypochondria hypocondrie *f*

hypochondriac (person) hypocondriaque *m/f*; malade *m/f* imaginaire

hypochondriac hypocondriaque *adj*.

hypodermic needle aiguille *f* pour piqûres

hypodermic syringe seringue *f* pour injections

hypoglycaemia (glucose deficiency in bloodstream) hypoglycémie *f*

hypotensive hypotensif -ive *adj*

hypothalamus (brain area controlling hunger, thirst, temperature etc.) hypothalamus *m*

hypothermia hypothermie *f*

hypothermia, induced hibernation *f* artificielle

hypothyroidism (subnormal activity of thyroid gland) hypothyroïdie *f*

hypotrophy (insufficiency in child growth/ development) hypotrophie *m*

hysterectomy hystérectomie *f*

hysteria hystérie *f*

hysterography (womb X-ray) hystérographie *f*

hysteric; hysterical person hystérique *m/f*

hysterical hystérique *adj*.

ice pack poche *f* de glace

icterus (jaundice) ictère *m*

idiocy idiotie *f*; imbécillité *f*

ileitis (inflammation of last portion of the intestine) iléite *f*

ileum (last portion of small intestine) iléon *m*

iliac (of the lower body or ilium area) iliaque *adj*

iliopsoas muscle (flexes the hip joint) psoas *m*; muscle *m* psoas-iliaque

ill mal *m* (*pl* -aux)

ill (of person) malade *adj.*

ill, gravely/seriously gravement malade

ill, to feel avoir mal *m* au cœur

illness maladie *f*

illness, harmless/mild maladie *f* benigne

illness, short and violent maladie *f* aiguë

illness, systemic (illness which spreads throughout the body, but with little known origin) maladie *f* systèmique

illness caused by a previous one (of) sécondaire *adj*

illness with no known cause (of) essential(le) *adj*

illness forming calcium deposits (of) calcifiant(e) *adj*

illness with physical cause maladie *f* somatique

illness in early pregnancy (of) tératogène *adj*

imaginary smells hallucination *f* olfactive

imbalance (between parts of anatomy usually same size eg. lungs, feet) déséquilibre *m*

imbecile imbécile *m/f*

imbecilic imbécile *adj*

imbecility imbécillité *f*

immersion syncope hydrocution *f*

immune defence system défenses *fpl* immunitaires

immune system système *m* immunitaire

immunity immunité *f*

immunity, acquired/ developed immunité *f* acquise

immunity, inborn immunité f naturelle

immunisation immunisation *f*

immunodeficiency déficience *f* immunitaire

immunologist immunologiste *m/f*; immunologue *m/f*

impaction (bone parts driven or wedged together and not moveable) impaction *f*

impairment of concentration, intelligence, memory asthénie *f* psychique

imperceptible with an ultrasound scan anéchogène *m*

impetigo (contagious skin infection) gourme *f*; impétigo *m*

implant (bone/skin or metal/ plastic to replace body part) implant *m*
implant, dental implant *m* (dentaire)
impotence impuissance *f*; impotence *f*
inability to breathe lying down orthopnée *f*
inability to move correctly (but not physically handicapped) apraxie *f*
inadequacy insuffisance *f*
incisor dent *f* incisive
inclining/reclining feature on para-medical armchair bascule *f* assise
incontinence incontinence *f*
incontinence pad couche *f* pour incontinents
incontinent incontinent(e) *adj*
increase, to (dose, etc.) majorer *v*
increase in majoration *f*
increasing dependence (on medicine/pill) accoutumance *f*
incubation incubation *f*
incubation period période *f* d'incubation
incubator couveuse *f*
incurable incurable *adj*
incurable person incurable *m/f*
incurably ill, the malades incurables
independent (physically) autonome *adj*
indication (medical or medicinal) indication *f*
indigestion indigestion *f*
indigestion (severe) crise *f* de foie
induced delivery accouchement *m* provoqué
industrial disease maladie *f* professionnelle
industrial hygiene hygiène *m* du travail
industrially disabled person invalide *m/f* du travail
infancy bas âge *m*; petite enfance *f*
infant care puériculture *f*
infantile paralysis paralysie *f* infantile
infarction (dead tissue through lack of blood) infarctus *m*
infect, to infecter *v*
infected, to become s'infecter *v*
infected infecté(e) *adj*

infected area for microscope examination coupe *f*
infection infection *f*
infection (through injury), accidental inoculation *f* accidentelle
infection, secondary surinfection *f*
infectious infectieux -euse *adj*
infectious disease maladie *f* infectieuse
infertility infertilité *f*
infestation infestation *f*
infest, to infester *v*
infiltration infiltration *f*
infirmary infirmerie *f*
infirmity infirmité *f*
inflammation/swelling fluxion *f*
inflammation medicines (group) corticoïde *m*
inflammatory inflammatoire *adj*
influenza; flu affection grippale *f*; grippe *f*
influenzal grippal(e) *adj*
influx influx *m*
infrared infrarouge *adj*
infrared radiation rayonnement *m* infrarouge
ingrowing nail ongle *m* incarné
inguinal (groin) hernia hernie *f* inguinale
inhalation inhalation *f*
inhale, to inhaler *v*
inhaler inhalateur *m*
inhaler, pocket-sized inhalateur *m* de poche *f*
inhibitor (natural substance or medicine) inhibiteur *m*
inhibitor of blood coagulation inhibiteur *m* de la coagulation
inhibitory inhibiteur -trice *adj*
initial incision area (in operation) abord *m*
injected injecté(e) *adj*
injection infiltration *f*; injection *f*; piqûre *f*
injection, to give an piquer *v*
injection, to have an se faire piquer *v*
injections (small) in or just under skin mésothérapie *f*
injure, to blesser *v*; léser *v*
injure oneself, to se blesser *v*
injury blessure *f*
inmate (mental hospital) interné(e)
inner ear cavity vestibule *m* de l'oreille interne

inoculate, to inoculer *v*
inoculation (injection of microbes) inoculation *f*
insanity démence *f*; folie *f*
insect bite piqûre *f* d'insecte
insect repellent lotion *f* contre les insectes
insemination, artificial insémination *f* artificielle
insemination, artificial (by donor) (AID) insémination *m* artificielle par donneur (IAD)
insensibility narcose *f*
inside intra- (as prefix)
insipid diabetes (deficiency of hormone regulating kidney) diabète *m* insipide
insomnia insomnie *f*
insomniac (person) insomniaque *m/f*
insomniac insomniac *adj*
instep cou-de-pied *m*
instillation (with drops for ear, eye, etc.) instillation *f*
institutional therapy (treatment over a period of time in a psychiatric home) thérapie *f* institutionnelle
institutionalise, to (patient) institutionnaliser *v*
institutionalised, to become s'institutionnaliser *v*
instructions (for taking medicine/pills) mode d'administration *f*
insufficiency; inadequacy (of an organ or set of organs to function properly which can lead to total failure) insuffisance *f*
insufficient natural growth development due to malnutrition hypotrophie *f*
insufflate, to (blow/breathe air, gas, powder into a body cavity) insuffler *v*
insufflation insufflation *f*
insulin insuline *f*
insulin-dependent person (requiring daily injections) or illness insulinodépendant(e) *m/f*
insulin-requiring person or illness (temporary) insulinorequérant(e) *m/f*
insulin injection injection *f* d'insuline
insulin treatment for diabetes traitement *m* par insuline

intelligence quotient (IQ) quotient *m* intellectuel (QI)

intensive care soins *mpl* intensifs

intensive care, to be in être *v* en réanimation

intensive care unit service *m* de la réanimation

interaction (adverse) of two medicines interaction *f* médicamenteuse

interferon (proteins released by cells) interféron *m* humain

interior interne *adj*

intermission intermission *f*

intermittent intermittente *adj*

internal interne *adj*

internal bleeding hémorragie interne *f*

internal illnesses (study of) médecine *f* interne

internal tissue swelling; gumma gomme *f*

interrupt, to (treatment, etc.) interrompre *v*

intervene, to (operate) intervener *v*

intervention intervention *f*

intestine intestin *m*

intestine, abnormal closing up of achalasie *f*

intestines, chronic inflammation of maladie *f* de Crohn

intestinal blockage blocage *m* intestinal; occlusion *f* intestinale

intestinal blockage signs syndrome *m* occlusif

intestinal flora (not an abnormal condition) flore *f* intestinale

intestinal transition transit *m* intestinal

intestinal wash lavage *m* d'intestin

intoxicate, to intoxiquer *v*

intracranial pressure hypertension *f* intracrânienne

intradermic injection injection *f* intradermique

intramuscular injection injection *f* intramusculaire

intraoculaire blood pressure tension *f* intraoculaire; pression *f* oculaire

intra-uterine coil sterilet *m*

intra-uterine contraceptive (IUD) dispositif *m* intra-utérin (DIU)
intravenous intraveineux -euse *adj* (IV)
intravenous injection injection *f* intraveineuse
intravenous X-ray of kidneys and urinary tracts urographie *f* intraveineuse
intubate, to intuber *v*
intubation intubation *f*; tubage *m*
invalid infirme *m/f*; malade *m/f*
invalid car voiture *f* pour handicapé
invasive (disease or procedure) invasif -ive *adj*
inversion/abnormal position of organ déviation *f*
invertebrate disc disque *m* intervertébral
involution (organ size reduction) involution *f*
iodine iode *m*; teinture d'iodine *f*
iodine base enema fluid (used in preparation for scanning the large intestine) lavement *m* à la Gastrograffine ®
ionising radiation radiation *f* ionisante
iridology (diagnosis by examination of iris) iridologie *f*
iris (of eye) iris *m*
iritis (iris inflammation) iritis *f*
iron fer *m*
iron, excess of in body (disease caused by) hémochromatose *f*
iron (concerning) martial(e) *adj*
iron deficiency déficit *m* en fer; carence *f* martiale
irradiation; radiation irradiation *f*
irreducible (of fractures, hernias) irréductible *adj*
irregular (of pulse, etc.) ondulant(e) *adj*
irrigate, to irriguer *v*
irrigation irrigation *f*
irrigator (hydrotherapeutic appliance to eliminate toxins in the intestines, vagina, etc) irrigateur *m*
irritable bowel syndrome colopathie *f* fonctionnelle; syndrome *m* de l'intestin *m* irritable
irritant irritant *m*

irritant irritant(e) *adj*
irritation irritation *f*
ischaemia (blood circulation blockage or disorder in an organ) ischémie *f*
isolation isolement *m*
isotonic solution (solution equal in molecular concentration to blood plasma) solution *f* isotonique
itch; itching démangeaison *f*
(the) itch (la) gale *f*
itch, to démanger *v*
itching, severe prurit *m*
itching, severe anal; anal pruritus prurit *m* anal
itching reduction/elimination product antiprurigineux *m*

jab, to (inject) piquer *v*
jaundice; icterus ictère *m*; jaunisse *f*
jaw mâchoire *f*
jaw, lower/upper mâchoire *f* inférieure/supérieure
jawbone maxillaire *m*
jawbone (concerning); maxillary maxillaire *adj*
jawbone, lower/upper maxillaire *m* inférieur/supérieur
jaw cavity setting for teeth alvéole *f* dentaire
jaw surgery chirurgie *f* maximillaire
jejunum (second part of small intestine) jéjunum *m*
jellyfish sting piqûre *f* de méduse
joint articulation *f*
joint, surgical repair of impaired arthroplastie *f*
joint blocking blocage *m* articulaire
joint displacement (off centre) excentration *f*
joints, blocked/paralysed (in flexed position) flessum/flexum *m*
joint, difficulty/inability to move a; ankylosis ankylose *f*
joints disorder algodystrophie *f* sympathique
jugular vein veine *f* jugulaire
junction (of two organs or organ parts) jonction *f*
juniper genévrier *m*

Kaposi's illness/sarcoma/ syndrome (malignant tumour syndrome) maladie *f*/ sarcome *m* de Kaposi
keep, to tenir *v*
keep out of children's reach ne pas laisser à la portée *f* des enfants
keep out of children's reach and view tenir *v* hors de la portée et de la vue des enfants
karyotype (number and chromosome types in a cell nucleus) caryotype *m*
keratin (fibrous proteins in hair) kératine *f*
keratitis (inflammation of the cornea) kératite *f*
keratosis (thickening of the cornea) kératose *f*
keyhole surgery to examine artery arthroscopie *f*
kidney rein *m*
kidney's ability to filter waste from the blood clairance *f*
kidney cancer cancer *m* du rein
kidneys are no longer producing urine anurie *f* vraie
kidneys block the urine fausse anurie *f*
kidney/renal failure défaillance *f* rénale; insuffisance *f* rénale
kidney/renal failure, acute défaillance *f* rénale; insuffisance *f* rénale aiguë
kidney and pelvis inflammation pyélonéphrite *f*
kidney inflammation; nephritis néphrite *f*
kidney machine rein *m* artificiel
kidney specialist néphrologue *m/f*
kidney stone calcul *m* rénal
kidney transplant greffe *f* de rein; transplantation *f* du rein
kinetics, heart (study of) cinétique *f* du coeur
kleptomania kleptomanie *f*
knead, to pétrir *v*
kneading massage pétrissage *m*
knee genou *m*
knee, back of jarret *m*
knee, back of (concerning) poplité(e) *adj*
knee, dislocated genou *m* déboîté
knee cartilage, deterioration of lésion *f* méniscale
knee pain; gonalgy gonalgie *f*

knee rheumatism gonarthrose *f*
knee support genouillère *f*
kneecap rotule *f*
kneecap, displaced excentration *f* de la rotule
knock-kneed genoux cagneux *mpl*

L-dopa (form of dopa: a treatment for Parkinson's disease) L-dopa *f*
labelling étiquetage *m*
labial (of lips) labial(e) (*pl* -aux) *adj*
labour, childbirth travail *m*
labour, difficult des couches *fpl* pénibles
labour pains douleurs *fpl* de l'accouchement
labour room chambre *f* de travail préparatoire à l'accouchement
laceration déchirure *f*; lacération *f*
Lachman's sign (tibia pulls forward or backward more than normal) signe de Lachman *m*
lachrymal lacrymal(e) (*mpl* -aux) *adj*
lachrymal (tear) glands glandes *fpl* lacrymales
lactation lactation *f*
lactobacilli (bacteria producing lactic acid) lactobacilli *mpl*
lactose (sugar in milk) lactose *m*
lance, to percer *v*
lancet (surgical knife) lancette *f*
lanoline lanoline *f*; graisse *f* de laine
laparotomy (stomach operation) laparotomie *f*
laparotomy, investigative laparotomie *f* exploratrice
large intestine gros intestin *m*
large intestine, first part of caecum *m*
large intestine, abnormal cavities in diverticulose *f* colique
large intestine, elongation of (not an illness) dolichocôlon *m*
large intestine, excessive air in; aerocoly aérocolie *f*
large intestine part sewn up after surgery poche *f*
large intestine parts forming a square cadre *m* colique

laryngectomy (removal of part or entire larynx) laryngectomie *f*

laryngitis laryngite *f*

laryngoscope (instrument) laryngoscope *m*

laryngoscopy (detailed inspection of larynx using a laryngoscope) laryngoscopie *f*

larynx larynx *m*

larynx inflammation with hard cough; croup croup *m*

laser laser *m*

laser beam rayon *m* laser

Lassa fever (acute tropical disease) fièvre *f* de Lassa

lassitude lassitude *f*

latent period (incubation period of illnress) temps *m* de latence

latex gloves gants *m* latex

laxative laxative *m*

laxative laxatif -ive *adj*

lead poisoning; saturnism saturnisme *m*

lead poisoning colic colique *f* de plomb *m*

leg jambe *f*

leg, broken jambe *f* cassée

leg, articulated jambe *f* articulée

leg, wooden jambe *f* de bois

leg, artificial jambe *f* artificielle

legs, strong/sturdy jarrets *mpl* d'acier

leg bone, lower and outer; fibula péroné *m*

leg-bone growing pain apophysite *f* tibiale antérieure

legionnaire's disease maladie *f* du légionnaire

lentigo lentigo *m*

leprosy lèpre *f*

lesion lésion *f*

lethal létal(e) (*mpl* -aux) *adj*

lethal dose dose *f* mortelle; dose *f* létale

lethal (possibly) combination of medicines, would cause lysis through a cell-destroying (lytic) process cocktail *m* lytique

lethargy léthargie *f*

leucocyte (white corpuscle) leucocyte *m*

leucoma (white opacity in the cornea) taie *f*

leucoplasy (abnormal white patch on tongue/genitals/ inside mouth) leucoplasie *f*
leuc(k)orrhea (vaginal discharge) leucorrhée *f*; pertes *f* blanches
leucotomy (surgery to white nerve fibres of brain) leucotomie *f*
leukaemia cancer du sang *m*; leucémie *f*
level (of sugar, alcohol, cholesterol, etc.) taux *m*
libido libido *f*
lice infestation pédiculose *f*
lie heavy on the stomach, to embarrasser *v* l'estomac
life expectancy espérance *f* de vie
life-saving lessons cours *mpl* de sauvetage
ligament ligament *m*
ligature (esp. in surgery) ligature *f*
ligature, to ligaturer *v*
light fever fébricule *f*
light massage effleurage *m*
light meal collation *f*
light therapy luminothérapie *f*
light therapy lamp, with protective screen lampe *f* de luminothérapie *f*, avec écran de protection
limb membre *m*
limb, lower/upper membre *m* inférieur/supérieur
limp claudication *f*, boiterie *f*
limp, to boiter *v*
line of vision/sight rayon *m* de vision *f*
lip lèvre *f*
lip, upper/lower lèvre *f* supérieure/inférieure
lip inflammation (corners) perlèche *f*
lip salve pommade *f* pour les lèvres
lipase (fat-breaking enzyme) lipase *f*
lipase level in blood lipasémie *f*
lipid (fatty acid/oils/wax/ steroid) lipide *m*
liposoluble (fat soluble) liposoluble *adj*
liposuction liposuccion *f*
liquorice réglisse *f*
listen to heartbeat/breathing, to (using ear or stethoscope) ausculter *v*

listeriosis (food-poisoning infection) listériose *f*

lithiasis (small stones in ducts, cavities and tubes) lithiase *f*

lithiasis (kidney stones causing inflammation) lithiase *f* rénale

liver foie *m*

liver (of the) hépatique *adj*

liver-coloured hépatique *adj*

liver complaint hépatopathie *f*

liver complaint sufferer hépatique *m/f*

liver disorder désordre *m* hépatique

liver failure insuffisance *f* hépatique

liver specialist hépatologue *m/f*

lobe, lower/middle/upper (lung) lobe *m* inférieur/moyen/supérieur (du poumon *m*)

lobotomy (pre-frontal brain lobe incision) lobotomie *f* cérébrale

local/topical (medicine/pain/anaesthetic) topique *adj*

local anaesthesia anesthésie *f* locale

location (of lesion) repérage *f*

lockjaw tétanos *m*

locum remplaçant(e) *m/f*

long and slender (of body shape) filiforme *adj*

long and slender (of finger) grêle *adj*

longevity longévité *f*

long-sightedness hypermétropie *f*; presbytie *f*

lordosis (inward curvature of the spine) lordose *f*

lose consciousness, to perdre *v* conscience

lose weight, to mincir *v*

lose weight quickly, to (informal) décoller *v*

loss/losing perte *f*

loss of consciousness perte *f* de connaissance

loss of hair chute *f* des cheveux

loss of memory perte *f* de mémoire

loss of sense of smell anosmie *f*

lotion lait *m*; lotion *f*

louse pou *m* (*pl* poux)

low-calorie foods/dishes cuisine *f* minceur

low-fat cooking cuisine *f* allégée/légère

low sperm count oligo-asthénospermie *f*
lumbago lombalgie *f*; lumbago *m*
lumbar lombaire *adj*
lumbar area région *f* lombaire
lumbar puncture ponction *f* lombaire
lumbar vertebrae vertèbres *fpl* lombaires
lump bosse *f*
lump (after a bump or wound) oedema *m* réactionnel
lump; tumour grosseur *m*
lunacy folie *f*; démence *f*
lung poumon *m*
lungs, difficult passage of air through syndrome *m* obstructif pulmonaire
lung cancer cancer *m* du poumon
lung cavity, permanent air bubble in bulle *f* dans le poumon
lung collapse, partial infarctus *m* pulmonaire
lung congestion congestion *f* pulmonaire
lung crepitations (crackling/rattling sound detected by stethoscope with certain lung diseases) crépitation *f* pulmonaire; râles *mpl* crépitants
lung (part of) disorder atélectasie *f*
lung inflammation alvéolite *f*
(the) lungs are affected (les) poumons *m* sont pris
lung X-ray aire *f* pulmonaire
lungs air capacity, measurement of (with spirometer) spirométrie *f*
lupus (ulcerous skin disease) lupus *m*
lupus erythematis, chronic lupus *m* érythémateux chronique
lupus erythematis, systemic (lupus infection throughout the body) lupus *m* érythémateux disséminé
lupus vulgaris (TB with dark red skin patches due to TB inoculation) lupus *m* vulgaire
lying down on the back position décubitus *m* dorsal
lying down on the front/stomach décubitus *m* frontal
lying down on the side décubitus *m* latéral

lying down position décubitus *m*

lymph (colourless fluid with only white corpuscles) lymphe *f*

lymph gland/node ganglion *m* lymphatique

lymph gland, swelling of; adenitis adénite *f*

lymph vessel vaisseau *m* lymphatique

lymphangitis (inflammation of lymphatic vessels) lymphangite *f*

lymphatic lymphatique *adj*

lymphatic system (network of vessels conveying lymph) système *m* lymphatique

lymphatic drainage drainage *m* lymphatique

lymphosarcoma (cancer of lymph gland/node tissue) lymphosarcome *m*

lysis (cell/bacteria destruction) lyse *f*

lysis, relating to/causing lytique *adj*

macrobiotic (Zen Buddhist dietary system) macrobiotique *adj*

macrobiotics macrobiotiques *fpl*

macroscopic (visible to the naked eye) macroscopique *adj*

macula (spot-like central area of retina) macule *f*

macula (dark spot in the skin) macule *f*

macular degeneration (deterioration of the most important part of the retina) dégénérescence *f* maculaire liée à l'âge (DMLA)

mad cow disease maladie *f* de la vache folle

madness démence *f*; folie *f*

magic mushroom champignon *m* hallucinogène

magnesium magnésium *m*

magnesium deficiency déficit *m* en magnésium

magnetic resonance imagery (MRI) imagérie *f* par résonance *f* magnétique (IRM)

magnetism (for rheumatism, lumbago, kidney stones,

etc.) magnétisme *m*; magnétothérapie *f*
magnifying glass loupe *f*
malaria malaria *f*; paludisme *m*
malarial fever fièvre *f* paludéenne
male menopause andropause *f*
malignancy malignité *f*
malignant (worsening/growing illness/tumour) malin(igne) *adj*
malingerer faux -sse malade *m/f*
malnutrition sous-alimentation *f*
Malta fever brucellose *f*
mammary mammaire *adj*
mammary abscess abcès *m* mammaire
mammary density (mammography factor) densité *f* mammaire
mammary glands glandes *fpl* mammaires
mammectomy mammectomie *f*
mammography (2D breast X-ray) mammographie *f*
mandible (jaw) mandibule *f*
mandible (of, concerning) mandibulaire *adj*
mania (serious mental disorder) manie *f*
manic depression psychose *f* maniocodépressive; cyclothymie *f*
manifest sign(s) of illness symptôme(s) *m* actif(s)
manipulation manipulation *f*
manipulation of the spine manipulation *f* vertébrale
manually-operated relaxation armchair/lounger fauteuil *m* de repos manuel
marasmus (emaciation due to nutritional deficiency) marasme *m*
marjoram (oil extract) origan *m*
mark (on body) trace *f*
mark on skin, brown tache *f* café au lait
marker (in blood tests, shows development or diminution of illness) marqueur *m*
marking (of product) étiquetage *m*
marrow moelle *f*
marrow, bone moelle *f* osseuse
massage massage *m*
massage, body percussion *f*
massage, cardiac massage *m* cardiaque
massage, kneading pétrissage *m*

massage, localised frictional frictions *fpl* localisées
massage, scalp massage *m* du cuir chevelu
massage, to masser *v*
massage, to have a se faire masser *v*
massage glove gant *m* de crin
massage lightly, to effleurer *v*
massage oil huile *f* de massage
masseur -euse masseur *m*, -euse *f*
massively obese (category in body weight index: see indice de masse corporelle in Fr-Eng section) obésité *f* massive
mastectomy (breast removal operation) mastectomie *f*
mastication mastication *f*
mastitis (breast inflammation) mastite *f*
mastoid process (protuberance on bone behind ear) mastoïde *f*
mastoid (conical shape) mastoïde *adj*
mastoiditis (inflammation of mastoid process) mastoïdite *f*
maternity department, ward service *m* d'accouchement, de maternité
matron surveillante *f* générale
matter matière *f*
mattress matelas *m*
maturation maturation *f*
maxillary (concerning jaw/jawbone) maxillaire *adj*
measles rougeole *f*
measure, to; measure out, to doser *v*
measurement of volumes (in certain organs) volumétrie *f*
mediate (medium for obtaining result) médiat(e) *adj*
medical médical(e) *adj*
medical analysis/blood tests laboratory laboratoire *m* d'analyses *fpl* médicales
medical box/cabinet armoire à pharmacie *f*
medical care soins *m* médicaux
medical certificate certificat *m* médical; attestation *f* médicale
medical check-up examen *m* médical
medical code of ethics déontologie *f* médicale

medical confidentiality secret *m* médical
medical consultant chef *m* de service
medical emergency urgence *f* médicale
medical examination examen *m* médical
medical fees honoraires *fpl* médicaux
medical file dossier *m* médical
medical imagery imagérie *f* médicale
medical imagery department service *m* d'imagérie médicale
medical imagery using gamma rays gammagraphie *f*
medical law droit *m* médical
medical needle aiguille *f*
medical supervision surveillance *f* médicale
medicated skin plaster/patch (such as nicotine patch) timbre *m* transdermique
medication for external use médicament *m* à usage externe
medicinal herb herbe *f* médicinale
medicine (study of) médecine *f*
medicine (medicament) médecine *f*; médicament *m*
medecine, alternative/non-conventional médecine *f* alternative/douce/naturelle
medicine, complementary médecine *f* parallèle
medicine, conventional médicament *m* allopathique
medicine, homeopathic (in small doses) médicament *m* homéopathique
medicine, preventive médecine *f* préventive
medicine, remedial médecine *f* curative
medicine, therapeutic substance *f* thérapeutique
medicine (study of effects on the body) pharmacodynamie *f*
medicine price sticker (used for social security reimbursement) vignette *f*
medicine, to take se soigner *v*
medicine ball (large exercise ball) médecine-ball *m*
medicine made up on prescription préparation *f* magistrale
meditation méditation *f*

medulla moelle *f*
medulla oblongata (spinal bulb at bottom of brain) bulbe rachidien *m*
medullary (relating to spinal cord) médullaire *adj*
megalomania mégalomanie *f*
melancholia mélancolie *f*
melancholic mélancolique *adj*
melanin (pigment, tanning under sun and/or UV rays) mélanine *f*
melanism (excessive melanin darkening the skin) mélanisme *m*
melanoma (tumour, usually malignant, from melanin-forming cells) mélanome *m*
membrane (covering certain organs) séreuse *f*
membrane, inflammatory couenne *f*
memory mémoire *f*
memory (of, concerning) mnésique *adj*
memory block blocage *m* de mémoire
memory lapse défaillance *f* de mémoire
memory (visual) loss apraxie *f*
Ménière's disease (circulation problem causing dizziness) vertige *m* de/maladie *f* de Ménière
meningitis méningite *f*
meningitis, the three symptoms of trépied *m* méningitique
meningitis, spinal méningite *f* cérébro-spinale
meningococcus (microbe causing some forms of meningitis) méningocoque *m*
meninx (membrane covering brain and other nervous system organs) méninges *f*
meninx tumour méningiome *m*
meniscus (rounded cartilage in knee) ménisque *m*
meniscus, of/concerning méniscal(e) (*mpl* -aux) *adj*
meniscus, surgical removal of ménisectomie *f*
menopausal ménopausique *adj*
post-menopausal ménopausée *adj*
menopause ménopause *f*
menopause process périménopause *f*

menorrhagia (abnormally long menstruation) ménorragie *f*
menstrual menstruel(le) *adj*
menstrual periods, absence of; amenorrhoea aménorrhée *f*
menstruation menstruation *f*; règles *f*
menstruation, total absence of (in adolescent girl) aménorrhée primaire *f*
menstruation, occasional absences of (in a patient who otherwise menstruates normally) aménorrhée *f* secondaire
'mental' age (based on IQ test results) âge *m* mental
mental block blocage *m*
mental confusion/disorder (temporary) confusion *f* mentale
mental defect déficit *m* intellectuel
mental deficiency débilité *f* mentale; faiblesse *m* mentale
mental fatigue surmenage *m* intellectuel
mental health santé *f* mentale
mental hospital hôpital *m* psychiatrique
mental illness maladie *f* mentale
mental retardation arriération *f* mentale
mental shock commotion *f* mentale
mental unbalance déséquilibre *m* mental
mental well-being bien-être *m* mental
mentally handicapped person déficient *m* -ente *f* mental(e); dégénéré(e) *m/f*
mentally ill person malade *m/f* mental(e)
mercury mercure *m*
mesencephalon (midbrain) mésencéphale *m*
metabolism métabolisme *m*
metacarpus (hand bone) métacarpe *m*
metal brace (for broken bone) fixateur *m* externe
metal material used for surgical implants matériel *m* métallique
metastasis (transfer of disease within the body) métastase *f*

metastasise, to métastaser *v*
metatarsus (foot bone) métatarse *m*
meteorism (air-inflated stomach and intestines) météorisme *m*
methylene blue antiseptic bleu de méthylène *m*
microbe microbe *m*
microbiologist microbiologiste *m/f*
microbiology microbiologie *f*
micturition (urination) miction *f*
midbrain mésencéphale *m*
middle-aged entre deux âges *adj*
mid-wife sage-femme *f*
mid-wife, male (rare) maïeuticien *m*
migraine migraine *f*
milk lait *m*
mind-expanding; 'mind-blowing' (of drug) hallucinogène *adj*
minipill minipilule *f*
minor complication complication *f* mineure
minute (fracture) a minima *adj*
miscarriage avortement *m* spontané; fausse couche *f*
mixed feeding allaitement mixte *m*
modification (of organ, following illness) remaniement *m*
moist dressing pansement *m* humide
moisturise skin, to hydrater *v*
moisturiser crème *f* hydratante
moisturising (skin) réhydratation *f*
moisturising hydratant(e) *adj*
molar (tooth) molaire *f*
mole (spot) grain *m* de beauté; lentigo *m*
moniliasis (see also thrush) moniliase *f*; candidose *f*
monitoring monitorage *m* (formal); monitoring *m* (colloquial)
mood humeur *f*
morning-after pill pilule *f* du lendemain
morning sickness nausées *fpl* matinales
morphine morphine *f*
morphology (general aspect/form of body/organs) morphologie *f*

mosquito repellent (product) antimoustique *adj*
motions selles *fpl*
motion, to have a/to pass a aller *v* à la selle
motionless, to remain/stay rester *v* sans bouger
motivity (normal mobility of body) motricité *f*
motor neuron neurone *m* moteur
motor nerve nerf *m* moteur
mountain sickness mal *m* de montagne
mouth (concerning); buccal buccal(e) *adj*
mouth, inside of the cavité *f* buccale
mouth-to-mouth (resuscitation) bouche-à-bouche *m*
mouth inhaler inhalateur *m* buccal
mouth inflammation; stomatitis stomatite *f*
mouth ulcer aphte *m*
mouthwash/mouth rinse bain *m* de bouche; eau dentifrice *f*
move around, to (person) se déplacer *v*
move around quickly, to se déplacer rapidement *v*
mucous muqueux -ueuse *adj*
mucous membrane muqueuse *f*
mucoviscidosis (pancreatic disease) mucoviscidose *f*
mucus glaire *f*
mud-bath bain *m* de boue *f*
multiple arthritis; polyarthritis polyarthrite *f*
multiple fractures fractures *fpl* multiples
multiple sclerosis sclérose *f* en plaques; sclérose *f*
multiple mumps oreillons *m*; parotidite *f* ourlienne
muscle muscle *m*
muscle, calf mollet *m*
muscle activity, examination of électromyogramme *m* (EMG)
muscle contraction (automatic reaction in reflex test) réflexe *m* ostéo-tendineux
muscle elasticity tonicité *f*
muscle (rotating) rotateur *m*
muscle wasting condition amyotrophie *f*
muscular musculaire *adj*

muscular dystrophy dystrophie *f* musculaire

muscular tissue tissu *m* musculaire

musculature (body/organs muscular system) musculature *f*

mushroom champignon *f*

mushroom, edible champignon *m* comestible

mushroom disease (following consumption of certain fungi) aspergillose *f*

mustard poultice cataplasme *m* de moutarde; cataplasme *m* sinapisé

mutagen (agent promoting genetic change) agent *m* mutagène

mutagenic mutagène *adj*

muteness mutité *f*

mutism (following psychological shock or mental illness) mutisme *m*

myasthenia gravis (rare chronic disease with muscular weakness) myasthenia *f*

mycology (study of fungi) mycologie *f*

mycosis (fungal disease) mycose *f*

mycotoxin (toxic substance produced by a fungus) mycotoxine *f*

myelitis (spinal cord inflammation) myélite *f*

myocarditis (heart inflammation diseases) myocardite *f*

myocardium (heart muscle) myocarde *m*

myoglobin (iron-content protein in muscle cells) myoglobine *f*

myopathy (progressive muscle atrophy) myopathie *f*

myopic (short-sighted) myope *adj*

myopia (short-sightedness) myopie *f*

myxoedema (thyroid disorder resulting in overweight, physical and mental lethargy) myxoedème *m*

naevus (birthmark) naevus *m*

nail ongle *m*

nail, split ongle *m* dédoublé

nails, fragile/brittle ongles *mpl* cassants
nails, well-manicured ongles *mpl* soignés
nail care soins *mpl* des ongles
nail clippers pince *f* à ongles
nail deformation hippocratisme *m* digital
nail file lime *f* à ongles
nail hardener durcisseur *m* d'ongles
nail scissors ciseaux *mpl* à ongles
nail varnish vernis *m* à ongles
nail varnish remover dissolvant *m*
nape of the neck nuque *f*
nappy couche *f* pour bébés
nappy, disposable couche *f* jetable; couche-culotte *f*
nappy rash érythème *m* fessier
nappy rash cream crème *f* contre les rougeurs *m*
narcolepsy (disease with fits of sleepiness) narcolepsie *f*
narcosis (insensibility) narcose *f*
narcotic narcotique *m*; stupéfiant *m*
narcotic narcotique *adj*
narrow passage between two bones/organs défilé *m*
narrow passage between first rib and clavicle défilé *m* costo-claviculaire
narrowing rétrécissement *m*
narrowing of aortic (heart) valve rétrécissment *m* aortique (RA)
narrowing of mitral (heart) valve rétrécissement *m* mitral (RM)
nasal nasal(e) *adj*
nasal cavity cavité *f* nasale
nasal inhalation (for administration of medicine) par voie *f* nasale
nasal instrument for withdrawal babies' mucus mouche-bébé *m*
nasal mucus (snot) morve *f*
nasal septum (between the nostrils) cloison *f* du nez *m*
nasal septum displacement déviation de la cloison *f* natale
nasty (attack of...) mauvais(e) *adj*
natural naturel(le) *adj*
natural childbirth parturition *f*
natural death mort *f* naturelle

natural medicine (exercise, massage, heat without medication); physiotherapy physiothérapie *f*

natural tendency to be right- or left-handed/footed latéralisation *f*

natural wearing down of body parts (e.g. cartilage) abrasion *f*

naturopathy (natural treatment: without medicines) naturopathie *f*: naturothérapie *f*

nausea nausée *f*

navel nombril *m*; ombilic *m*

neck cou *m; col m*

neck area inside mouth (around teeth and gums) collet *m*

neck bone, second axis *m*

neck, stiff raideur de la nuque *f*; torticolis *m*

neck of the bladder col *m* de la vessie

neck pain cervicalgie *f*

neck and groin pulses pouls *m* centraux

neck rest travel cushion coussin *m* de voyage

neck vertebrae arthrosis uncarthrose *f*

necrosis (death of body tissue or part) nécrose *f*

needle (such as syringe) aiguille *f*

negative (results) négatif -ive *adj*

neonatal neonatal(e) *adj*

neonatal period période *f* néonatale

nephritis (kidney inflammation) néphrite *f*

nephrosis (chronic kidney disease) néphrose *f*

nerve nerf *m*

nerve centre centre/point *m* névralgique

nerve cluster at end of spinal cord queue *f* de cheval

nerve cluster at end of spinal cord, symptoms caused by crushed syndrôme *m* de la queue de cheval

nerve inflammation; neuritis névrite *f*

nerve root racine *f* nerveuse

nerve root, of/concerning radicumaire *adj*

nerve tumour gliome *m*; neurinome *m*
nervous nerveux -euse *adj*
nervous breakdown dépression *f* nerveuse
nervous person neurotonique *f*
nervous tension nervosité *f*
nervous shock choc *m* nerveux
nervous system système *m* nerveux
nervousness nervosité *f*
nervy nerfs *m* à vif (colloquial)
nettle rash urticaire *f*
neural (of nerve or nervous system) neural(e) (*mpl* -aux) *adj*
neuralgia névralgie *f*
neuralgia running from neck down the arm névralgie *f* cervico-brachiale
neuralgic névralgique *adj*
neurasthenia (depression) neurasthénie *f*
neurasthenic (person) neurasthénique *m/f*
neurasthenic neurasthénique *adj*
neuritis (nerve inflammation) névrite *f*
neuroleptic (sedative) neuroleptique *m*
neuroleptic neuroleptique *adj*
neurological neurologique *adj*
neurologist neurologue *m*
neurology neurologie *f*
neuroma (tumour) névrome *m*
neuromuscular (concerning nerves and muscles) neuromusculaire *adj*
neuron (nerve cell) neurone *m*
neuron, motor neurone moteur *m*
neuronal neuronal(e) *adj*
neurosis névrose *f*
neurosis, obsessional/phobic névrose *f* obsessionnelle/phobique
neurotic névrotique *adj*
neurotic depression dépression *f* névrotique
neutralise, to (pain) neutraliser *v*
new-born baby nouveau-né *m* -née *f*
new-born (unweaned) baby nourrisson *m*
nicotine addiction nicotinisme/nicotisme *m*; tabagisme *m*
nicotine patch patch *m* à la nicotine

nicotine poisoning nicotinisme/nicotisme *m*
nightmare cauchemar *m*
nipple mamelon *m*
nocturnal (of fever, symptoms, occurrence etc.) horaire *f* nocturne
nodule (small swelling or lump) nodule *m*
'no mortal danger' bulletin (for patient) 'jours ne sont pas en danger'
node nodus; nodosité
node, lymph ganglion *m* lymphatique
noises, harmful sons *m* nocifs (90–120dB)
non-conventional medicine médecine *f* alternative/douce/naturelle
noradrenaline (hormone causing nerve or muscle impulse) noradrénaline *f*
normal normal(e) (*mpl* -aux) *adj*
normal-sized de dimension *f* normale
normal weight poids *m* normal (see also indice de masse corporelle in French-English section)
nose nez *m*
nose, blocked nez *m* bouché
nose, dripping goutte *f* au nez
nose, inflammation of; rhinitis rhinite *f*
nose, stuffy nez *m* pris
nose drops gouttes *fpl* pour le nez
nosebleed saignement de nez *m*
nosebleeding; epistaxis épistaxis *f*
nosecaps filtres *m* nasaux
nosocomial (of infectious illnesses contracted in hospitals, clinics, surgeries) nosocomial(e) (*mpl* -aux) *adj*
nostril narine *f*
not serious discrét -ète *adj*
nourishing nutritif -ive *adj*
nuclear magnetic resonance imaging (MRI) imagerie par résonance magnétique nucléaire *f*; (IRM)
nucleus noyeau *m*
nulligest (woman who has never been pregnant) nulligeste *f*
numbness engourdissement *m*
numeration numération *f*
nurse infirmier *m* -ère *f*

nurse, charge/head surveillant(e) *m/f;* infirmière *f* en chef
nurse, district infirmier/ère visiteur/euse *m/f*
nurse, home garde-malade *m/f*
nurse, self-employed state registered infirmier/ère *m/f* diplômé(e) d'état en libéral
nurse, state registered infirmier/ère *m/f* diplômé(e) d'état
nurse, visiting infirmier/ère *m/f* visiteur/euse
nurse's aide aide-soignant(e) *m/f*
nursery nurse puéricultrice *f*
nursery nursing puériculture *f*
nursing home maison *f* de retraite; résidence *f* médicalisée
nursing sister infirmière *f* chef
nutrition nutrition *f*
nutritional nutritionnel(le) *adj*
nutritional report (for a patient) bilan *m* nutritionnel
nutritive nutritif -ive *adj*
nystagmus (rapid, unintentional eye movements) nystagmus *m*
obese obèse *adj*
obesity obésité *f* (see also indice de masse corporelle in French-Eng section)
objective (of symptom which can be objectively verified/measured) objectif -ive *adj*
observation observation *f*
observation (e.g. clinical) constatation *f* clinique
observation, to be/to put under être/mettre *v* en observation
obsessional eating (overeating) hyperphagie *f*
obsessive compulsive disorder (OCD) trouble *m* obsessionnel compulsif (TOC)
obstetric(al) obstétrique; obstétrical(e) *adj*
obstetric clinic clinique *f* obstétrique
obstetric department service *m* d'obstétrique *f*
obstetrician obstétricien (ne) *m/f*
obstetrics obstétrique *f*
obstruct, to engorger *v*; obstruer *v*
obstruct (artery), to oblitérer *v*

obstruction obstruction *f*; engorgement *m*
occipital area (rear of the skull) région *f* occipitale
occipital bone, of/concerning occipital(e) *adj*
occiput (back of the head) occiput *m*
occlude, to (block or close up pores or orifice) occlure *v*
occlusion occlusion *f*
occupational disease maladie *f* du travail
occupational therapist ergothérapeute *m/f*
occupational therapy ergothérapie *f*
oculist (eye specialist) oculiste *m/f*
odontology (dentistry) odontologie *f*
oedema (dropsy) œdème *m*
oedematous allergic reaction (with swollen face and possibly the throat) œdème *m* de Quinke
Oedipus complex complexe *m* d'Œdipe
oesogastrectomy (surgical removal of part of gullet and stomach) oesogastrectomie *f*
oesophagus (gullet) œsophage *m*
oestrogen (female hormone) œstrogène *m*
oesophagus, inflammation of oesophagite *f*
oil; lipid lipide *m*
ointment remède *m*
ointment for haemorrhoids remède *m* hémorroïdaire
ointment for skin pommade *f*
old age vieillesse *f*
olecranon (elbow bone) olécrâne *m*
olfaction (sense of smell) olfaction *f*
olfactory hallucination hallucination *f* olfactive
oliguria (reduced urination capacity) oligurie *f*
oncogene (gene which can transform a cell into a tumour cell: present in tobacco smoke) oncogène *m*
onychomycosis (fungal disease affecting nails) onychomycose *f*
ooze out, to écouler *v*

open fracture fracture *f* ouverte
open-heart surgery opération *f* à coeur ouvert
operate, to intervenir *v*; opérér *v*
operated on, patient who has been opéré(e) *m/f*
operating theatre bloc *m* opératoire; salle *f* d'opération; théâtre *m* d'opérations
operation intervention *f*; opération *f*
operation, to have an se faire opérér *v*
operation without overnight hospitalisation opération *f* ambulatoire
opthalmia (eye inflammation) ophtalmie *f*
ophthalmic optician, ophthalmologist ophtalmologiste *m/f*; ophtalmologue *m/f*
ophthalmology (general) ophtalmologie *f*
ophthalmology (concerning spectacle and contact, lenses) contactologie *f*
opiate (a sedative) opiat *m*
opposing muscles, organs or systems antagonistes *fpl*
ophthalmia (eye inflammation) ophtalmie *f*
optician, dispensing opticien *m* -ienne *f*
optic nerve nerf *m* optique
oral oral(e) (*mpl* -aux) *adj*
oral cavity cavité *f* buccale
oral hygiene hygiène *f* bucco-dentaire
orally oralement *adv*
orally, to be taken (for administration of medicine) par voie buccale/orale *f*
orbit orbite *f*
orchitis (testicle inflammation) orchite *f*
organ organe *m*
organ, abnormally opaque (on X-rays) hyperdense *adj*
organ, functional failure of défaillance *f*
organ, inversion or abnormal position of déviation *f*
organ, part of secteur *m*
organ, surgical operation to remove ablation *f*; exérèse *f*
organ collapse or stop in growth aplasie *f*
organ containing too much blood, of congestif -ive *adj*

organ faintly discernible on X-rays (a sign that it no longer functions) exclu(e) *adj*
organ growth, first stages of germe *m*
organ malfunction trouble *m* trophique
organ transplant greffe *f* d'organe
organ, to remove an prélever *v* un organe
organic product produit *m* bio
organism organisme *m*
organs (normally) immediately adjacent accolement *m*
orthodontics (teeth straightening) orthodontie *f*
orthopaedic orthopédique *adj*
orthopaedic appliance appareil *m* orthopédique
orthopaedic equipment, to fit a disabled person with appareiller *v*
orthopaedic and traumatic wounds surgery chirurgie *f* orthopédique et traumatique
orthopaedic exercises gymnastique *f* orthopédique
orthopaedics orthopédie *f*
orthopist (eye-movement therapist) orthoptiste *m/f*
Osgood's disease (leg growing pains) maladie *f* d'Osgood
ossification (the process of becoming bone) ossification *f*
osteitis (bone inflammation or bone disease) ostéite *f*
osteoarthritis (degenerative disease of the joints) arthrose *f*; ostéoarthrite *f*
osteomalacia (lack of bone calcium) ostéomalacie *f*
osteomyelitis (bone or bone marrow inflammation) ostéomyélite *f*
osteopath ostéopathe *m/f*
osteopathy ostéopathie *f*; médecine *f* manuelle
osteophyte (abnormal shape/ extension to bone on edge of rheumatic joint) lipping *m*; ostéophyte *m*
osteoporosis (brittle and fragile bones) ostéoporose *f*
osteosarcoma (bone cancer) ostéosarcome *m*
osteosclerosis (abnormal bone thickening) ostéosclérose *f*

otitis (ear inflammation/ infection, of outer/inner ear) otite *f* (externe/interne)
otology (study of ear diseases) otologie *f*
otorhinolaryngology (study and treatment of ear, nose and throat conditions) oto-rhino-laryngologie *f*
outer pulses (wrists, temple etc.) pouls *mpl* périphériques
outgrowth excroissance *f*
out-of-true (bone) désaxé(e) *adj*
outpatient malade *m/f* ambulatoire
outpatient examinations examens *mpl* en externe
outpatient treatment traitement *m* ambulatoire
out-turned (limb) valga *adj*
ovarian cyst kyste *m* de l'ovaire
ovarian follicle follicule *m* ovarique
ovary ovaire *m*
ovary or testicle gonade *f*
ovaries, removal of annexectomie *f*
overcome, to (illness) surmonter *v*
overdose surdosage *m*; surdose *f*
(esp. drugs) overdose *f*
(a mistakenly administered injection with potential fatal results, shortly after a previous injection with the same product) injection *f* déchaînante
overeat, to se suralimenter *v*
overeating suralimentation *f*
overeating disorder (anorexia-bulimia) anorexie-boulimie *f*
overexertion surmenage *m* physique
overheat, to échauffer *v*
overheating (of blood) échauffement *m*
overtaxed brain cerveau *m* fatigué
oversized trop grand(e); énorme; gigantesque *adj*
overweight surpoids *m*
overworked heart coeur *m* fatigué
ovulate, to ovuler *v*
ovulation ovulation *f*
ovum (cell) ovule *f*
oxygen oxygène *m*

oxygen or carbon dioxide level measurement in the blood saturométrie *f*
oxygen cylinder/bottle bouteille *f* d'oxygène
oxygen mask masque *m* à oxygène
oxygen passage to blood (in the lungs); alveolus alvéole *f* pulmonaire
oxygen tent tente *f* à oxygène
oxygen treatment oxygénothérapie *f*
oxyuriasis (pinworm/threadworm illness) oxyurose *f*

pacemaker pacemaker *m*; stimulateur *m* cardiaque; stimulateur *m* artificiel
pack (surgical/medical dressing) mèche *f*
pack (open wound) with gauze, to mécher *v*
pad tampon *m*
pads under the fingers/roll of flesh bourrelet *m* de chair
paediatric nurse (in a hospital) puéricultrice *f*
paediatric care puériculture *f*
paediatrician pédiatre *m/f*
paediatrics pédiatrie *f*
Paget's cancer of the nipple maladie *f* cutanée de Paget
Paget's bone deformation disease maladie *f* osseuse de Paget
pain douleur *f*
pain, acute douleur *f* aiguë
pain, constant douleur *f* persistante
pain, dull douleur *f* sourde
pain, intermittent douleur *f* intermittente
pain, nagging douleur *adj* irritante
pain, sharp douleur *f* aiguë; élancement *m*
pain, shooting élancement *m*
pain, throbbing douleur *f* lancinante
pain, (of/concerning) local/topical topique *adj*
pain-alleviating care soins *mpl* palliatifs
pain in the arm brachialgie *f*
pain in middle of the stomach douleur *f* épigastrique

pain, violent and sudden facial névralgie *f* faciale; névralgie *f* du trijumeau
painful douloureux -euse *adj*
painful joints arthralgie *f*
painkiller calmant *m* antidouleur; analgésique *m*
painless indolore *adj*
pain-relieving antidouleur *adj*
pain-relieving (clip on) electrodes électrodes *f* pour les douleurs
pain relieving medicines, over-the-counter (not usually reimbursed, even if prescribed) médicament *m* de comfort
pain-relieving product, medical produit *m* du confort médical
pain-relieving/palliative treatment for terminally ill traitement *m* palliatif
pain threshold seuil *m* de la douleur
palate palais *m*
palate, cleft palais *f* fendu
pale, to look avoir *v* une petite figure/petite mine
paleness pâleur *f*
palliative palliatif -ive *adj*
palliative care soins *mpl* palliatifs
pallor pâleur *f*
palm paume *f*
palpate, to (to examine medically by touch) palper *v*
palpation (medical examination, by touch) palpation *f*
palpitations palpitations *fpl*
palsy, with uncontrollable tremors paralysie *f*
palsy, cerebral paralysie *f* cérébrale
palsy, shaking paralysie *f* agitante
paludism paludisme *m*
pancreas pancréas *m*
pancreas, end of queue *f* du pancréas
pancreas calcification disease maladie *f* pancréatique calcifiante
pancreatitis (pancreas inflammation) pancréatite *f*
pancreatic pancréatique *adj*
pancreatic disease; mucoviscidosis mucoviscidose *f*

panty liner protège-slip *m*
papille (small button-like protuberance of organ or body part) papille *f*
papilloma (small and harmless growth) papillome *m*
papule or papula; pimple papule *f*
papulo-pustole (pimple containing pus) papulo-pustule *f*
paracetomol paracétamol *m*
paralyse, to paralyser *v*
paralysed down one side (of body); hemiplegic hémiplégique *adj*
paralysed down one side (of body), person; hemiplegic hémiplégique *m/f*
paralysed joints, in flexed position flessum/flexum *m*
paralysed man or woman paralyse(ée) *m/f*
paralysis paralysie *f*
paralysis of half the body syndrome *m* pyramidal
paralysis of one side of the body; hemiplegia hémiplégie *f*
paralytic (person) paralysé(e) *m/f*
paramedic auxiliaire *m/f* medical(e)
paramedical paramedical(e) *adj*
paranoia paranoïa *f*
paraplegia paraplégie *f*
paraplegic paraplégique *adj*
paraplegic man/woman paraplégique *m/f*
parasite parasite *m*
parasitic(al) parasitique; parasitaire *adj*
parasitic flatworm douve *f*; distome *m*
parasympathetic nervous system (from brain to lower spinal cord) système *m* parasympathique
parathyphoid paratyphoïde *adj*
parathyphoid fever fièvre *f* parathyphoïde; paratyphoïde *f*
parathyroid parathyroïde *adj*
parathyroid gland parathyroïde *f*
paresis (partial paralysis) parésie *f*
parietal (concerning the wall of the body or any of its cavities) pariétal(e) (*mpl* -aux) *adj*

parietal pain in the chest/ribs (not the heart) douleur *f* pariétocostale
Parkinson's disease maladie *f* de Parkinson
parotiditis (saliva gland inflammation) parotidite *f*
paroxysm (crisis point/ climax) paroxysme *m*
part of the anatomy corps *m*
partially sighted person malvoyant(e) *m/f*
parturien (about to give birth) parturiente *adj*
pass (exceed), to dépasser *v*
pass on/away, to partir *v*
pass on an illness, to communiquer *v* une maladie
pass out, to tomber *v* dans les pommes (informal)
passive smoking (inhalation of other people's cigarette smoke) tabagisme *m* passif
patch test patch-test *m*
patella (kneecap) rotule *f*
pathogen (causing disease) agent *m* pathogène
pathogenic pathogène *adj*
pathological pathologique *adj*
pathological haemolysis (abnormal elimination of red corpuscles) hémolyse *f* pathologique
pathological laboratory laboratoire *m* pathologique
pathologist (disease specialist) pathologiste *m/f*
pathology pathologie *f*
pathology, anatomy and cytology (study of cells) anatomie *f* et cytologie *f* pathologiques
patient malade *m/f*; patient(e) *m/f*
patient, post-operation opéré(e) *m/f*
patient, severely ill grand(e) malade *m/f*
patient, terminally ill condamné(e) *adj*
patient affected by cyanosis cyanosé(e) *m/f*
patient who is no longer feverous, of apyrétique *adj*
patient with coronary artery disorder coronarien(ne) *f*
patient discharge (release from hospital) sortie *f*

paunch, to have a/to be developing a avoir *v*/prendre *v* du ventre

pause (between two courses of treatment); temporary pause in a treatment intercure *f*

peach-like complexion peau de pêche *f*

pectoral pectoral(e) (*mpl* pectoraux) *adj*

pectoral (chest) muscle, greater muscle *m* grand pectoral

pectoral girdle ceinture *f* scapulaire

pectoral muscle pectoral *m* (*pl* -aux)

pediculosis (lice infestation) pédiculose *f*

pellagra (disease due to vitamin deficiency) pellagre *f*

pellet grain *m*

pelvis bassin *m*; pelvis *m*

pelvis and kidney inflammation pyélonéphrite *f*

pelvis, inflammation of; pyelitis pyélite *f*

pelvis, lower petit bassin *m*

pelvic (bone) girdle ceinture *f* pelvienne

penicillin pénicilline *f*

penis pénis *m*; verge *f*

penis, inflammation of tip of balanite *f*

pepsin (enzyme in gastric juice) pepsine *f*

peptic (concerning or promoting digestion) peptique *adj*

peptic ulcer ulcère *m* peptique; ulcère *m* de l'estomac

period(s) flux *m* menstruel(s); période *f* menstruelle

peppermint plant menthe *f* poivrée

percuss, to percuter *v*

percussion (body tapping as part of diagnosis) percussion *f*

percussion massage tapotement *m*

percutaneous (through the skin) percutané(e) *adj*

perforate, to perforer *v*

perforation perforation *f*

perfume parfum *m*

perfusion perfusion *f*

periarthritis (inflammation of ligaments and tendons

surrounding a joint) périarthrite *f* scapulo-humérale

pericardium (heart's membraneous sac) péricarde *m*

pericarditis (pericardium inflammation) péricardite *f*

perineum (area between anus and scrotum or vulva) périnée *f*

period (menstruation) règles *fpl*

periodic périodique *adj*

peripheral nervous system système *m* nerveux périphérique

peristalis (automatic digestive movements) péristaltisme *m*

peritoneum (serum-producing stomach membrane) péritoine *m*

peritoneum, of/concerning peritoneal(e) (*mpl* -aux) *adj*

peritoneum, advanced stage of a stomach cancer which extends to the carcinose *f* péritonéale

peritonitis (peritoneum inflammation) péritonite *f*

pernicious pernicieux -euse *adj*

pernicious anaemia anémie *f* pernicieuse progressive

peroxide peroxyde *m*

persecution mania délire *m* de persécution

personal hygiene hygiène *f* corporelle

personal medical records dossier *m* médical personnel (DMP)

personality disorder trouble *m* du caractère

personality test test *m* de personnalité

perspiration sudation *f*; sueur *f*; transpiration *f*

perspiration, slight perspiration *f*

pertussis (whooping cough) vaccine vaccin *m* contre la coqueluche

pessary (womb support/ contraceptive) ovule *m* (pharmacie); pessaire *m*

phagocytosis (ingestion of bacteria through the white corpuscles) phagocytose *f*

phalanx (finger bone) phalange *f*

phantom pregnancy grosseuse *f* nerveuse

pharmaceutical form (including packaging) forme *f* pharmaceutique

pharmaceutical product produit *m* pharmaceutique

pharmacist pharmacien(ne) *m/f*

pharmacology pharmacologie *f*

pharmacy pharmacie *f*

after hours (duty) pharmacy pharmacie de garde *f*

pharyngitis (pharynx inflammation) pharyngite *f*

pharynx (membrane-lined cavity behind the mouth and nose) pharynx *m*

phase phase *f*

phial flacon *m*

phimosis (foreskin constriction) phimosis *m*

phlebitis (inflammation of veins) phlébite *f*

phlegm glaire *f*

phobia phobie *f*

phosphorus phosphore *m*

photophobia (aversion to light) photophobie *f*

photosensitisation (reaction to light) photosensibilisation *f*

phrenic nerve (relating to the diaphragm) nerf *m* phrénique

physical examination; physical examen *m* fonctionnel

physical and psychological anxiety angoisse *f*

physical well-being bien-être *m*

physician médecin *m*

physiological haemolysis (natural elimination of red corpuscles) hémolyse *f* physiologique

physiological laboratory laboratoire *m* physiologique

physiological serum/ salt solution sérum *m* physiologique/artificiel

physiology physiologie *f*

physiotherapist; physio; physical therapist kinésithérapeute *m/f*; abbrev. kiné

physiotheraputic exercise exercice *m* de rééducation

physiotherapy kinésithérapie *f*; rééducation *f*

phytotherapy (herbal medicine) phytothérapie *f*

pia mater (innermost membrane around brain and spinal cord) pie-mère *f* (*pl* pies-mères)
pigeon-toed condition hallux valgus *m*
pigment pigment *m*
pigmentary retinitis (congenital condition leading to blindness) rétinite *f* pigmentaire
pigmentation pigmentation *f*
piles; haemorrhoids hémorroïdes *fpl*
pill pilule *f*; cachet *m*; comprimé *m*
pill, small grain *m*
pill, the (contraceptive) la pilule *f* contraceptive
pill box pilulier *m*
pimple bourgeon *m*; bouton *m*; papule *f*
pimple containing pus papulo-pustule *f*
pimply boutonneux -euse *adj*
pin (support) broche *f*
pinch pincement *m*
pinch, to pincer *v*
pinch mark pinçon *m*
pinna (outer part of ear) pavillon *m* de l'oreille
pinning (of fractured bone) brochage *m*
pinprick piqûre d'épingle *f*
pins and needles acroparesthésie *f*; formication *f*; fourmillement *m*
pinworm; oxuryid oxyure *m*
pipette compte-gouttes *m*
pituitary pituitaire *adj*
pituitary gland (at base of brain) glande *f* pituitaire; hypophyse *f*
pityriasis (flaking skin condition) pityriasis *m*
place point *m*
placebo placebo *m*
placenta placenta *m*
placenta, detachment of (from uterus) décollement *m* du placenta *m*
plague peste *f*
plasma plasma *m*
plasma bank banque *f* de plasma
plaster emplâtre *m*; plâtre *m*
plaster, adhesive pansement *m* adhésif

plaster, blister pansement *m* pour l'ampoule
plaster, corn emplâtre *m* pour les cors
plaster, hermetically sealed pansement *m* occlusive
plaster, to put/set in mettre *v* dans le plâtre
plaster bandage bande *f* plâtrée
plaster bandage providing support, wet appareil *m* plâtré
plaster cast gouttière *f*
plastic surgeon chirurgien(ne) *m/f* plastique
plastic surgery plastie *f*; chirurgie *f* plastique
plastic reconstruction/repair surgery chirurgie *f* plastique/ reconstructrice
platelets (for coagulation) plaquettes *f*
pleura (membranes lining thorax and over lungs) plèvres *mpl*
pleura (of/concerning thorax and lung membranes) pleural(e) (*pl* -aux) *adj*
pleural cavity cavité *f* pleurale
pleurisy pleurésie *f*
pleuritic pleurétique *adj*
plexus (nerve network) plexus *m*
plexus, solar plexus solaire *m*
pneumococcus (bacteria causing pneumonia and other infections) pneumocoque *m*
pneumoconiosis (dust-in-the-lungs disease) pneumoconiose *f*
pneumogastric nerve nerf *m* pneumogastrique
pneumology pneumologie *f*
pneumonia fluxion de poitrine *f*; pneumonie *f*
point point *m*
point (tip) pointe *f*
poison poison *m*
poison, to empoisonner *v*; intoxiquer *v*
poison treatment centre centre *m* anti-poison
poison specialist; toxicologist toxicologue *m/f*
poisoning empoisonnement *m*; intoxication *f*
poisonous mushroom champignon *m* vénéneux

poliomyelitis (infantile paralysis) paralysie *f* infantile *f*; poliomyélite *f*

poliomyelitis vaccine vaccin *m* de poliomyélite

pollution pollution *f*

polyarthritis (multiple arthritis) polyarthrite *f*; rhumatisme *m* déformant

polymyositis (rare muscle disease) polymyosite *f*

polyneuritis (nervous disorder) polynévrite *f*

polyp; polypus (small internal growth) polype *m*

polyp(s), surgical removal of polypectomie *f*

polyunsaturated (fat/oil molecule) poly-insaturé(e) *adj*

polyvalent polyvalent(e) *adj*

poor health, to be in avoir *v* une petite santé

porphyria (rare hereditary blood disease) porphyrie *f*

portal vein (to the liver) veine *f* porte

positive (results) positif -ive *adj*

positive result, falsly (second test advisable) résultat *m* faux positif

posterior rugae (cleft between the buttocks) raie *f* des fesses

post-menopausal ménopausée *adj*

postnatal postnatal(e) *adj*

postnatal depression dépression *f* post-partum; bébé blues *m* (informal)

postnatal fever (due to uterine infection) fièvre *f* puerpérale

postnatal pain tranchées *fpl* utérines

post-operative post-opératoire; (abbrev.) postop *adj*

post-operative depression dépression *f* opératoire

post-operative illness maladie *f* opératoire

post-operative shock choc *m* opératoire

post-partum (period immediately following childbirth) post-partum *m*

posture posture *f*

potassium potassium *m*

potassium level in the blood kalilémie *f*

Pott's disease (TB of the spine) mal *m* de Pott

potty pot *m* d'enfant

pouch separating different body organs capsule *f*

poultice cataplasme *m*

powder poudre *f*

practise, to pratiquer *v*

practitioner (GP or specialist) praticien(e) *m/f*

precautions before use (medicines) précautions *fpl* d'emploi

precision and concentration, patient's lack of désorganisation *m* (d'un malade)

precocious; early (of diagnosis) précoce *adj*

pre-eclampsia (pregnancy condition) prééclampsie *f*

pre-examination/pre-operation nerves (of patient) trac *m*

pregnant enceinte *adj*

pregnant with twins enceinte *f* de jumeaux *mpl* -elles *fpl*

pregnancy grossesse *f*; (strictly medical) gestation *f*

pregnancy, ectopic (fœtus outside womb) grossesse *f* extra-utérine

pregnancy, high-risk grossesse *f* à haut-risque

pregnancy termination for medical reasons avortement *m* thérapeutique

pregnancy test test *m* de grossesse

prehension (gripping) ability préhension *f*

pre-marital examination (for marriage settlement contracts) examen *m* prénuptial

premature baby premature(e) *m/f*

premature birth accouchement *m* prématuré

premature decline in hearing presbyacousie *f* précoce

premenstrual syndrom (PMS) syndrome *m* prémenstruel (PMS)

prenatal clinic clinique *f* prénatale

pre-operative préopératoire *adj*

preparation of patient before investigation or surgery préparation *f*

prepare someone (medically) for transport, to appareiller *v* un patient

prepuce (foreskin) prépuce *m*

prescribe, to (written) ordonner *v*

prescribed date date *f* prescrite

prescribed dose dose *f* prescrite

prescription, verbal prescription *f*

prescription, written ordonnance *f*

presentation (child delivery position) présentation *f*

pressure pression *f*

pressure point point *m* de compression *f*

prevention prévention *f*

preventive medicine médecine *f* préventive

previous personal or family (medical) history antécédent m (médical)

priapism (persistent erection) priapisme *m*

primary (of symptoms) primaire *adj*

prion (proteinous infection particle: associated with Creutzfeldt-Jakob disease) prion *m*

private bed (hospital room) lit *m* privé

prick one's finger, to se piquer *v* le doigt

probe (action of) sondage *m*

probe (instrument) sonde *f*

probe, to sonder *v*

probing sondage *m*

proboscis appendice *m* nasal

product produit *m*

product which checks bleeding astringent *m* and *adj*

progesterone (steroid hormone in the uterus) progestérone *f*

prognosis pronostic *m*

prognosis, reserved prognostic *m* réservé

progressive/worsening nature (of illness) évolutivité *f*

progressively destroys (relating to illness/disease) érosif -ive *adj*

prolapse (slipping forward/ down of a part/organ of body) prolapsus *m*

prolapse of an organ descente *f* d'organe
prolapse of the womb descente *f* de matrice
prolongation of life by medical intervention, uncomfortable acharnement *m* thérapeutique
prominent saillant(e) *adj*
pronation (forearm or hand) pronation *f*
properties (characteristics) propriétés *fpl*
properties, therapeutic propriétés *fpl* thérapeutiques
prophylaxis (preventive treatment) prophylaxie *f*
prostate gland prostate *f*
prostate gland, of/concerning prostatique *adj*
prostate operation, to have a se faire opérer *v* de la prostate
prostate cancer cancer *m* de la prostate
prostate tumour (benign) adénome *m* prostatique
prostatectomy (partial/total prostate gland removal) prostatectomie *f*
prostatitis prostatite *f*
prosthesis prothèse *f*
prosthesis placed inside the body endoprothèse *f*
protect oneself, to se protéger *v*
protein protéine *f*
protein content in the blood, excessive hyper-albuminémie *f*
protein content in blood, insufficient hypo-albuminémie *f*
protein substance in blood albumine *f*
protein enriched hyperprotidique *adj*
protuberance éminence *f*
protruding saillant(e) *adj*
protruding part of bone apophyse *f*
provide with medical care, to médicaliser *v*
pruritus (severe itching) prurit *m*
psittacosis (contagious bird disease) psittacose *f*
psoriasis (skin condition) psoriasis *m*
psychiatric psychiatrique *adj*
psychiatric disorder trouble *m* psychiatrique

psychiatric hospital hôpital *m* psychiatrique
psychiatrist psychiatre *m/f*
psychiatrist for the elderly gérontopsychiatre *m/f*
psychiatry psychiatrie *f*
psychiatry, child and adolescent psychiatrie *f* de l'enfant *m* et de l'adolescent *m*
pscychoanalysis psychanalyse *f*
psychoanalyst psychanalyste *m/f*
psychological psychologique *adj*
psychological defect déficit *m* psychologique
psychological shock choc *m* psychologique
psychological test test *m* psychologique
psychologist psychologue *m/f*
psychology psychologie *f*
psychometric (divination quality or feature) psychométrique *adj*
psychometric tests tests *mpl* psychométriques
psychopath psychopathe *m/f*
psychopathic psychopathe *adj*
psychopathy psychopathie *f*
psychosis psychose *f*
psychosomatic (of physical illness caused or worsened by mental stress) psychosomatique *adj*
psychotherapy psychothérapie *f*: (abbrev.) thérapie *f*
puberty puberté *f*
pubic pubien(ne) *adj*
pubic hair poils *mpl* du pubis
pubis pubis *m*
puerperal (caused by childbirth) puerperal(e) *adj*
puerperal fever (postnatal fever due to uterine infection) fièvre *f* puerpérale
puffy, to become gonfler *v*
puffy eyes yeux *m* gonflés
pull out, to extraire *v*
pulled (muscle) élongation *f*
pulmonary pulmonaire *adj*
pulmonary embolism embolie *f* pulmonaire
pulmonary lesion lésion *f* pulmonaire
pulmonary oedema (water-filled lungs) œdème *m* du poumon
pulmonary vein veine *f* pulmonaire

pulp (tooth) cavity cavité *f* pulpaire
pulsation pulsation *f*
pulse pouls *m*
pulse, to take the prendre *v* le pouls
pulse, abnormally slow; bradycardia bradycardie *f*
pulse blockage bloc *m* cardiaque
pulse irregularity intermittence *f*
pulse rate fréquence *f* cardiaque
puncture ponction *f*
pupil (eye) pupille *f*
pure ethyl alcohol alcool *m* absolu éthylique
purgation purgation *f*
purgative purgatif *m*; purge *f*
purgative purgatif -ive *adj*
purge purgatif *m*; purge *f*
purge, to purger *v*
purification épuration *f*
purpura (purple skin rash) purpura *m*
pus pus *m*
pus, containing purulent(e) *adj*
pustule pustule *f*
pustulosis pustulose *f*
put in splints, to éclisser *v*
put (someone) on a drip, to alimenter *v* au goutte-au-goutte
put on weight, to grosser *v*
put out a joint, to se déplacer *v* une articulation
PUVA therapy/treatment (with UV rays) puvathérapie *f*
pyelitis (pelvis inflammation) pyélite *f*
pylorus (stomach opening to small intestine) pylore *m*
pylorus inflammation antre du pylore *m*
pylorus stricture (condition in babies) rétrécissement *m* du pylore
pylorus stricture, operation to widen pyloroplastie *f*
pyrogenic (producing body heat or fever) pyrogène *adj*
pyrorrhoe (shrinking of gums and loosening of teeth) pyorrhée *f* alvéolaire
pyrosis (gastric acid return in the throat) pyrosis *m*

quadriplegic; tetraplegic (person with total limb paralysis) tétraplégique *m/f*

quadriceps femoris (thigh) muscle quadriceps *m* (femoral)
quadriplegia (paralysis of all four limbs) quadriplégie *f*
quarantine quarantaine *f*
quarantine, to put into mettre *v* en quarantaine
quivering (of flesh etc.) palpitant(e) *adj*
quivering movement (e.g. heart) fibrillation *f*

rabies rage *f*
(anti)rabies vaccination vaccination *f* antirabique
rachialgy (spinal column pain) rachialgie *f*
rachitis (rickets) rachitisme *m*
rachitic; concerning a rickets sufferer rachitique *adj*
radius bone, of/concerning radial(e) (*mpl* -aux) *adj*
radiant (spreading) irradiant(e) *adj*
radiation irradiation *f*
radioactive radioactif -ive *adj*
radioactivity radioactivité *f*
radiochemical laboratory laboratoire *m* radiochimique
radiography; X-ray photography radiographie *f*; radio *f*
radiological examination examen *m* radiologique
radiologist radiologue/radiologiste *m/f*
radiology radiologie *f*
radioscopy (X-ray examination of objects opaque to light) radioscopie *f*
radiotherapist radiothérapeute *m/f*
radiotherapy (radiation treatment) radiothérapie *f*
radius (arm bone) radius *m*
rage, to fly into a piquer *v* une colère *f*
rale (abnormal breathing sound) râle *m*
rape viol *m*
rape, to violer *v*
rare disease maladie *f* rare
rash éruption *f*
rattling noise crépitation *f*
Raynaud's syndrome (poor blood circulation) syndrome *m* de Raynaud; maladie *f* de Raynaud
reaction réaction *f*

reaction (extreme, possibly life-threatening to an antigen) anaphylaxie *f*
readjust, to réadapter *v*
receding récessif -ive *adj*
recipient receveur *m*; receveuse *f*
recipient, universal receveur *m* universel; receveuse *f* universelle
recommendations, doctor's prescription *f*
recommend, to conseiller *v*
reconstruction surgery chirurgerie *f* réparatrice
recording of several precisely measured medical tests polygraphie *f*
recover, to récupérer *v*
recovery guérison *f*; récupération *f*
rectal rectal(e) (*pl* -aux) *adj*
rectal inflammation; rectitis rectite *f*
rectal phial ampoule *f* à usage rectal
rectal probe toucher *m* rectal
rectoscope rectoscope *m*
rectoscopy (internal examination of the rectum with rectoscope) rectoscopie *f*
rectum rectum *m;* canal *m* anal
rectum and colon inflammation recto-colite *f*
rectum and colon inflammation with large intestine bleeding recto-colite *f* hémorragique
rectum, through the (for administration of medicine) par voie *f* rectale
recuperation récupération *f*
recuperate, to récupérer *v*; recouvrer *v*
recuperate from, to se rétablir *v* de
recur, to récidiver *v*
recurrence (of illness) récidive *f*
recurrent recurrent(e) *adj*
recurring (after complete recovery) récidivant(e) *adj*
recurring (illness or fever) périodique *adj*
recurring nature récidivité *f*
red blotch/patch rougeur *m*
red corpuscle érythrocyte *m*; globule *f* rouge; hématite *f*
red corpuscles, abnormally large macrocytose *m*

red corpuscles, dimunition of déglobulisation *f*
red corpuscles, reduction in number of anémie *f* hypochromique
red corpuscles and iron deficiency in the blood, reduction in number of anémie *f* hyposidérémique
red-corpuscle sedimentation speed vitesse de sédimentation globulaire *f* (VS)
red spots taches rouges *f*
redness of the skin exanthème *m*; rougeur *m*
red-skin infection; erysipelas éryipèle *m*
red skin, cream for crème *f* antirougeurs
reducible (fracture) réductible *adj*
reduction/setting (of fracture) réduction *f*
re-educate, to (limb) rééduquer *v*
reflex, automatic (in response to doctor's reflex test) réflexe *m* ostéo-tendineux
reflexology (massage through reflex points) réflexologie *f*
reflux (return of liquid in the body) reflux *m*
reflux of blood from liver to jugular vein reflux *m* hépato-jugulaire
reflux of urine from bladder to kidneys reflux *m* vésico-urétéral
refund remboursement *m*
regain one's strength, to recouvrer *v* ses forces
regain consciousness, to reprendre *v* conscience
regeneration (tissues/cells) régénération *f*
regenerative régénérateur -trice *adj*
regime régime *m*
regression régression *f*
regurgitation régurgitation *f*
rehabilitate, to rééduquer *v*
rehabilitation rééducation *f*
rehabilitation centre centre *m* de rééducation
rehabilitation therapy, to have/undergo faire *v* de la rééducation
reimbursement remboursement *m*

rejection (of graft/transplant) rejet *m*
relapse rechute *f*
relapse, to rechuter *v*
relapse, to have a avoir/faire *v* une rechute
relaxant relaxant *m*
relaxation détente *f*; relaxation *f*
relaxation drug décontractant *m*
relaxation therapy sophrologie *f*
relaxing relaxant(e) *adj*
relieve, to soulager *v*
relieve congestion, to décongestionner *v*
remain, to rester *v*
remain motionless/silent, to rester *v* sans bouger *v*/sans rien dire *v*
remedial gymnastics gymnastique *f* corrective
remedial indication indication *f* thérapeutique
remedial medicine médecine *f* curative
remedy médicament *m*; remède *m*
remission; abatement rémission *f*
remittance intermittence *f*
remittent (of fever) remittent(e) *adj*
remove hair from, to épiler *v*
remove surgically, to enlever *v*
removing plaster déplâtrage *m*
renal rénal(e) *adj*
renal dialysis dialyse *f* rénale; hémodyalise *f*
renal/kidney colic colique *f* néphrétique
renal/kidney failure défaillance *f* rénale; insuffisance *f* rénale
renal/kidney failure, acute défaillance *f* rénale; insuffisance *f* rénale aiguë
reopen, to (cut, etc.) raviver *v*
repetitive strain injury trouble *m* musculosquelettique
replacement (doctor) remplaçant(e) *m/f*
repletion (e.g. of stomach) réplétion *f*
rescue sauvetage *m*
resection (surgical removal of section/part of organ) résection *f*
resembling eczema eczématiforme *adj*
resolve, (remove) to résoudre *v*

reabsorb, to (liquid/surgical thread) résorber *v*
respiration respiration *f*
respiration, artificial respiration *f* artificielle
respirator réanimateur *m*; respirateur *m* artificiel
respiratory respiratoire *adj*
respiratory allergy allergie *f* respiratoire
respiratory difficulties, severe détresse *f* respiratoire
respiratory disease, acute maladie *f* aiguë de l'appareil respiratoire
respiratory failure arrêt *m* respiratoire
respiratory system système *m* respiratoire
respiratory tract appareil *m* respiratoire
respiratory ventilation ventilation *f* respiratoire
rest, to se reposer *v*
restless legs syndrome (RLS) restless legs syndrome (sometimes said in English); syndrome *m* des jambes sans repos (SJSR)
restoration (of dislocated bone/joint to proper position) recentrage *m*
resuscitate, to réanimer *v*; ranimer *v*
resuscitation réanimation *f*
resuscitator réanimateur *m*
retractor (muscle) écarteur *m*
retention rétention *f*
retina rétine *f*
retina, detachment of décollement *m* de la rétine
retinal diseases (other than retinitis) rétinopathie *f*
retinitis (retina inflammation) rétinite *f*
retrograde ejaculation (into bladder) éjaculation *f* rétrograde
retroverted (e.g. of the womb) rétroversé(e) *adj*
retrovirus (including the Aids virus) rétrovirus *m*
revulsion (counterirritation treatment) révulsion *f*
revulsive révulsif -ive *adj*
Rhesus/RH factor facteur *m* Rhésus
rhesus (RH) positive/negative rhésus *m* positif/négatif

rheumatic pains douleurs *f* rhumatismales
rheumatic rhumatismal(e) (*mpl* -aux) *adj*
rheumatism rhumatisme *m*
rheumatism, articular/joint rhumatisme *m* articulaire
rheumatism, back dosarthrose *f*
rheumatism and cramp (muscular pains) myodynie *f*
rheumatism cushion, heated and magnetised cousin *m* chauffant rhumatisme
rheumatism of the knee gonarthrose *f*
rheumatoid rhumatoïde *adj*
rheumatoid arthritis polyarthrite *f* rheumatoïde (PR); polyarthrite *f* chronique évolutive (PCE); rhumatisme *m* chronique articulaire
rheumatologist rhumatologiste *m/f* (abbrev. rhumato)
rheumatology (arthritis and rheumatism) rhumatologie *f*
rhinitis (nose inflammation) rhinite *f*
rhinopharyngitis (sore nose and throat) rhinopharyngoite *f* (abbrev. rhino)
rib côte *f*
rib, broken côte *f* cassée
rib or chest ache douleur *f* pariétocostale
rib cage cage *f* thoracique; gril *m* costal
rib cavity cavité *f* pleurale
riboflavin (vitamin B) riboflavine *f*
ribonucleic acid (controls body's protein composition) acide *m* ribonucléique
ribs côtes *fpl*
ribs, crushed enfoncement *m* de la cage thoracique
rickets rachitisme *m*
rickets, to have être *v* rachitique
rigor mortis rigidité *f* cadavérique
ringing in ears bourdonnement *m* d'oreilles *f*
rings under the eyes cernes *m*
ringworm (fungal skin infection) herpès *m* circiné; teigne *f*
rinsing solution solution *f* de rinçage *m*
rise in (increase) majoration *f*

Risser's growth chart (from birth to maturity) score/test *m* de Risser
rod (rod shaped structures in the eye) bâtonnet *m*
roll of fat bourrelet *m* de graisse *f*
roof of the mouth voûte/palatine *f* du palais
root racine *f*
rosacea (red acne) rosacée *f*; couperose *f*
rosemary (tonic) romarin *m*
roseola (rosy rash) roséole *f*
rotator (muscle) rotateur *m*
rotative (of muscle) rotateur *adj*
round-sholdered dos *m* rond
rounded end of long bone épiphyse *f*
roundworm ascaride *f*
roundworm disease ascaridiase/-iose *f*
royal jelly (vitamin product) gélée royale *f*
rubella (German measles) vaccine vaccin *m* contre la rubéole
ruinous pernicieux -euse *adj*
runny nose goutte *f* au nez
rupture éventration *f*; hernie *f*; rupture *f*
rupture, accidental solution *f* de continuité
rupture of aorta (main artery) dissection *f* aortique
rupture/tearing of tendon rupture *f* tendineuse
rusk biscuit *m* pour bébé

saccharin saccharine *f*
saccharose saccharose *m*
sacrum (bone between the two hip bones) sacrum *m*
safety glasses, goggles lunettes *fpl* de sécurité, de protection
safety helmet casque *m* de sécurité
safety pin épingle *f* de sûreté
safety razor rasoir *m* mécanique; rasoir *m* de sécurité
sage (salvia: healing plant) sauge *f*
sagittal suture (bone junction on top of skull) gouttière *f* sagittale
saliva salive *f*
saliva gland inflammation; parotiditis parotidite *f*

salivary glands glandes *f* salivaires

salmonella salmonella *f*; salmonelle *f*

salmonella food poisoning salmonellose *f*

salpingectomy (surgical removal of Fallopian tubes) salpingectomie *f*

salpingitis (inflammation of Fallopian tube or the Eustachian [ear] tube) salpingite *f*

sample (of blood, stools, etc.) prélèvement *m*

sample, blood: the taking of a blood sample prise *f* de sang

sample, to take a prélever *v* un échantillon

sampling prélèvement *m*

sanatorium sanatorium *m*

sanitary sanitaire *adj*

sanitary towel serviette *f* hygiènique

saphenous (leg) vein; saphena saphène *f*

sarcoidosis (disease resembling TB) sarcoïdose *f*

sarcoma (malignant tumour) sarcome *m*

SARS (severe acute respiratory syndrome) SARS (syndrome *m* respiratoire aigu sévère)

saturnism (lead poisoning) saturnisme *m*

sauna sauna *m*

scab croûte *f*

scabby scabieux -euse *adj*

scabies gale *f*

scald brûlure *f* d'eau bouillante *f*

scald, to ébouillanter *v*

scald oneself, to s'ébouillanter *v*

scale (skin) squame *f*

scalp cuir chevelu *m*

scalp massage massage *m* du cuir chevelu

scalpel scalpel *m*

scaly squameux -euse *adj*

scaly skin disease dermatose *f* squameuse

scan, to have a passer *v* un scanner *m*/scanographe *m*

scan ultrasonically, to échographier *v*

scanner (not necessarily medical) scanner *m*; scanneur *m*

scanner (exclusively medical) scanographe *m*; tomodensiomètre *m*
scanning tomodensitométrie *f*; scanographie *f*
scans scanographie *f*
scapula (shoulder blade) omoplate *f*; scapulaire *m*
scapular scapulaire *adj*
scar cicatrice *f*; stigmate *m*; trace *f*
scar tissue tissue *m* cicatriciel
scarificator (scalpel for small incisions) scarificateur *m*
scarify, to scarifier *v*
scarlet, to go piquer *v* un fard
scarlet fever scarlatine *f*
Scheuermann's disease (deformation of spinal column) maladie *f* de Scheuermann
schizophrenia schizophrénie *f*
schizophrenic schizophrène *adj*
scent parfum *m*
sciatic sciatique *adj*
sciatica sciatique *f*
sciatic nerve nerf *m* sciatique
scintigraphy (2D medical imagery using gamma rays) scintigraphie *f*
sclera (white of the eye) sclérotique *f*
sclerodermia (chronic skin and tissue hardening) sclérodermie *f*
sclerosis sclérose *f*
sclerotic, to become se scléroser
sclerotic sclérotique *adj*
scoliosis (curvature of the spine) déviation *f* de la colonne; scoliose *f*
scoliosis (to the left) scoliose *f* sinistroconvexe
scoliosis (to the right) scoliose *f* dextroconvexe
scorbutic (affected with scurvy) scorbutique *adj*
scotch test (biological test in anal area) scotch-test *m*
scored (of tablet) sécable *adj*
scrape, to racler *v*
scraper curette *f*
scratch éraflure *f*
screen, to dépister *v*
screening test dépistage *m*
screening test (for Aids) dépistage *m* pour le Sida
scrofula (condition with glandular swellings) scrofule *f*

scrotal scrotal(e) *adj*
scrotum bourses *f*; scrotum *m*
scrotum veins, expansion/widening of varicocèle *f*
scrub gommage *m*
scrub (massage), body gommage *m* du corps
scrub, facial gommage *m* du visage
scurf peau *f* morte
scurvy scorbut *m*
seasickness mal de mer *m*
seawater therapy cure *f* de thalassothérapie
seaweed algues *fpl*
seaweed bath bain *m* d'algues *fpl*
seaweed, product containing (used in thalassotherapy) produit *m* aux algues *fpl* laminaires
sebaceous (fatty: of skin) sébacé(e) *adj*
sebaceous cyst kyste *m* sébacé; loupe *f*
sebaceous gland glande *f* sébacée
seborrhea (excessive discharge of sebum) séborrhée *f*
sebum (sebaceous glands secretion) sébum *m*
secondary infection surinfection *f*
secretion sécrétion *f*
sectioned (of infected body part) area for microscope examination coupe *f*
sedation sédation *f*
sedative calmant *m* tranquillisant; psychotrope *m*; sédatif *m*
sedative sédatif -ive *adj*
sedentary sédentaire *adj*
sediment sédiment *m*
sedimentation sédimentation *f*
seeing things hallucination *f* visuelle
seep, to écouler *v*
self-destruct, to se nécroser
self-produced; autogenous autogène *adj*
seltzer (mineral) water; soda water eau *f* de Seltz
semen; sperm sperme *m*
semence semence *f*
semi- (meaning one side of) hémi- *prefix*
seminal (of/concerning semen) séminal *adj*

senile sénile *adj*
senility sénilité *f*
sensation sensation *f*
sense sens *m*
sense of smell odorat *m*; olfaction *f*
sense of smell, to have a keen avoir *v* l'odorat fin
sensitive sensitif -ive *adj*
sensitivity acuité *f*; sensibilité *f*
sensitisation sensibilisation *f*
sensitised sensibilisé(e) *adj*
sensory nerve (brain) nerf *m* sensitif
septic (fever/bacteria) septique *adj*
septic (wound) infecté(e) *adj*
septic, to become s'infecter *v*
septicaemia (septic poisoning) septicémie *f*
septicity septicité *f*; état *m* septique
septum (body partition) septum *m*
septum, nasal cloison *f* du nez
septum, of/concerning septal(e) *adj*
serenity sérénité *f*
serious grave *adj*
serious critical condition état *m* critique sévère
seriously ill gravement malade *adj*
seriously ill person grand(e) malade *m/f*
serology (tests for blood disease symptoms) sérologie *f*
seronegative (negative blood test result) séronégatif -ive *adj*
seropositive (positive blood test result) séropositif -ive *adj*
serotonin (compound in blood platelets and serum acting as neurotransmitter); drug group aiding sleep and depressive disorders sérotonine *f*
serous (containing serum) séreux -euse *adj*
serum sérum *m*
session (exercise, treatment) séance *f*
set, to (a fractured bone) consolider *v;* réduire *v*
seton (surgical cotton for wound drainage) séton *m* à mèche
setting (of fracture) consolidation *f*

setting (reduction of fracture) réduction *f*
setting (of limb, bone) pose *f* d'un plâtre
severe acute respiratory system (SARS) syndrome *m* respiratoire aigu sévère (SRAS)
severely disabled person grand invalide *m* civil
sew up, to suturer *v*
sex (genital) sexe *m*
sex, possessing a (sexual) sexué(e) *adj*
sex therapist sexologue *m/f*
sexless/asexual (person) asexué(e) *adj*
sexual sexuel(le) *adj*
sexual abstinence continence *f*
sexuality sexualité *f*
sexually transmitted disease (STD) maladie *f* sexuellement transmissible (STD)
shadow on the lung voile *m* au poumon
shake, to trembler *v*
shaking tremblement *m*
shaking palsy paralysie *f* agitante
shampoo shampooing *m*
shampoo, fortifying treatment shampooing/shampoing *m* traitant fortifiant
sharp aigu(ë) *f*
shave, to raser *v*
shin bone tibia *m*
shin bone, edge of crête *f* du tibia *m*
shingles herpès zosta *m*; zona *m*
shingles, of/concerning zostérien(ne) *adj*
shingles affecting eye and part of face zona *m* ophtalmique
shiver frisson *m*
shiver, to frissonner *v*; grelotter *v*; trembler *v*
shock (reaction, possibly fatal) choc (médical) *m*
shock due to anaesthetics choc *m* anaesthétique
shock due to sudden drop in blood pressure choc *m* hypovolémique *m*
shock, to chequer *v*
short-sighted myope *adj*
short-sightedness myopie *f*
shoulder épaule *f*
blocked/frozen shoulder épaule *f* bloquée

shoulder, fragile/easily dislocated instabilité *f* gléno-humérale
shoulder blade scapulaire *m*
shoulder end of the humerous bone tête *f* de l'humérus *m*
shoulder muscle; deltoid deltoïde *m*
shoulder muscle tendons coiffe *f* des rotateurs *mpl*
shrinking rétrécissement *m*
shuffling gait steppage *m*
shunt (surgical creation of alternative passage for blood circulation) shunt *m*
shunt, surgical (surgically created passage for blood flow directly from artery to vein) shunt *m* artério-veineux
sibilant sibilant(e) *adj*
(car) sick, to feel avoir *v* mal au cœur *m* en voiture *f*
sick, to feel avoir *v* mal au cœur *m*
sick leave congé *m* de maladie
sick person malade *m/f*
sickness maladie *f*
sickness, feeling of malaise *f*
side effects effets *mpl* secondaires
sight test examen *m* de la vue
sight testing chart tableau *m* d'acuité visuelle
sigmoid colon (penultimate part of large intestine) côlon *m* pelvien; sigmoïde *m* (abbrev. of colon *m* sigmoïde)
sigmoid colon, of/concerning sigmoïde *adj*
sigmoidectomy (removal of sigmoid colon) sigmoïdectomie *f*
significant significatif -ive *adj*
silicon silicone *f*
silicosis (miners' lung disease) silicose *f*
sinew tendon *m*
single-use only à usage unique *m*
sinus sinus *m*
sinusitis sinusite *f*
sinusitis infection with inflammation of the ethmoid ethmoïdite *f*
siphon siphon *m*
skeleton squelette *f*
skin peau *f*
skin, damaged peau *f* lésée
skin, dry peau *f* sèche

skin, dryness of the sécheresse *f* cutanée

skin, greasy peau *f* grasse

skin, hard durillon *m*

skin, loose/slack peau *f* relâchée

skin, through the; percutaneous percutané(e) *adj*

skin allergy allergie *f* cutanée

skin allergy, manifesting redness and blisters érythrodermie *f* bulleuse

skin bank banque *f* de peau

skin blister bulle *f* dermatologique

skin cancer cancer *m* de la peau

skin de-pigmentation; vitiligo vitiligo *m*

skin disease/burn from too much sunlight lucite *f* (see also sunbathing in this section and **capital soleil** in French-Eng section)

skin disease/dermatosis following consumption of non-edible fungus dermatophytose *f*

skin graft greffe *f* de peau

skin or sub-cutaneous injections mésothérapie *f*

skin inflammation; dermatitis dermatite *f*; dermite *f*

skin layer, excessive growth of hyperacanthose *f*

skin ointment pomade *f*

skin peeling treatment (usually laser) peeling *m*

skin protectors (body and head hair, finger and toe nails) phanères *mpl*

skin redness and fatty scabs on baby dermite *f* séborrhéique du nourrisson

skin sensitivity to touch or to heat, abnormal paresthésie *f*

skin specialist; dermatologist dermatologiste *m/f*

skin test cuti-réaction *f*

skin test, positive reaction to (symptoms are present) virage *m* d'une cuti-réaction

skull boîte *f* crânienne; crâne *m*

skull bone behind the nose cornet *m*

sleep sommeil *m*

sleeping/sleepiness, frequent/ prolonged hypersomnie *f*

sleeping pill somnifère *m*

sleeping sickness maladie *f* du sommeil

sleepwalk, to marcher *v* en dormant; être *v* somnambule
sleepwalker somnambule *m/f*
sleepwalking somnambulisme *m*
sleep therapy cure *f* de sommeil
slender mince *adj*
slenderness minceur *f*
slim mince *adj*
slim, to maigrir *v*
slimming amincissant *adj*
slimming course cure *f* d'amaigrissement *m*
slimming diet régime *m* minceur; régime *m* amaigrissant
slimness minceur *f*
sling (arm) écharpe *f*
slipped disc hernie *f* discale
slowing down (physical or organ functions) ralentissement *m*
small of the back chute *f* des reins
small-of-the-back cushion support coussin *m* de positionnement dos
smallpox variole *f*
small intestine intestine *m* grêle
small intestine, excessive air in aéroiléie *f*
small intestine, inflammation of; enteritis entérite *f*
small therapeutic doses doses *fpl* homéopathiques
smear frottis *m*
smear, blood frottis *m* sanguin
smear, cervical frottis *m* cervico-vaginal
smell (scent), to sentir *v*
smoking addiction tabagisme *m*; dépendance *f* tabagique
smooth onctueux -euse *adj*
snakebite serum sérum *m* antivenimeux
sneeze éternuement *m*
sneeze, to éternuer *v*
sneezing éternuement *m*
snore, to ronfler *v*
snoring ronflement *m*
snot morve *f*
snow-blindness ophtalmie *f* des neiges
snow glasses lunettes *fpl* de glacier
soap savon *m*
soap, household savon *m* de Marseille
soap, 100 per cent vegetable content savon *m* 100 per cent végétal

soap, liquid savon *m* liquide
soap, toilet savon *m* de toilette
soapy water eau *f* savonneuse
socket, bone cavité *f* articulaire
soda water eau *f* de Seltz
sodium bicarbonate bicarbonate de sodium *m*
sodium free désodé(e) *adj*
soft mou *m* molle *f adj*
soft parts of body parties *fpl* molles
soft drug drogue *f* douce
soft tissue part of lung, kidney and other organs parenchyme *m*
soften, to ramollir *v*
softening ramollissement *m*
softener lotion, skin adoucissant *m*
solar plexus plexus solaire *m*
sole plante *f* (du pied *m*)
sole inflammation aponévrosite *f* plantaire
soluble soluble *adj*
soluble tablet cachet *m* soluble
solution solution *f*
solution soluté *m*
solution form, in en solution *f*
solvent dissolvant *m*
somatic somatique *adj*
soothing (cream, etc.) apaisant(e) *adj*
soothing émollient(e) *adj*; tranquillisant(e) *adj*
soothing agent émollient *m*
soporific somnifère *m*
soporific soporifique *adj*
sore plaie *f*
source of infection foyer *m* de l'infection
spa station *f* thermale
spa course of treatment cure *f* thermale
spa-water spray/spa-water atomiser vaporisateur *m*; eau *f* thermale
space between two bones (used in X-ray readings) interligne *f*
sparkling (mineral) water eau *f* gazeuse
spasm contracture *f*; spasme *m*
spasms, involuntary facial and arm spasmophilie *f*
spasms, involuntary violent series of spasme *m* clonique
spasmodic croup faux croup *m*
spatula spatule *f*
spatula section linking arm to chest acromion *m*

specialist spécialiste *m/f*
spectacles lunettes *fpl* de vue
speculum (surgical inspection instrument) speculum *m*
speech difficulty trouble *m* du langage
speech disorder dysarthrie *f*
speech, total/partial loss of (or ability to understand); aphasia aphasie *f*
speech therapy orthophonie *f*; rééducation *f* de la parole
speedy prompt(e) *adj*
speedy recovery prompt rétablissement *m*
sperm semence *f*; sperme *m*
sperm bank banque *f* de sperme
sperm count and analysis spermogramme *m*
spermatic cord (nerves, ducts, blood vessels going to the testicles) cordon *m* spermatique
spermatic weakness (linked to male sterility) asthénospermie *f*
spermicidal spermicide *adj*
spermicide spermicide *m*
sphincter sphincter *m*
sphygmomanometer (instrument that measures blood pressure) sphygmomanomètre *m*; tensiomètre *m* electronic
sphygmomanometer, wrist sphygmomanomètre *m* électronique de poignet
spina bifida spina bifida *m*
spina bifida, mild spina-bifida *m* occulta
spinal/vertebral column rachis *m*
spinal column colonne *f* vertébrale
spinal column pain; rachialgy rachialgie *f*
spinal cord cordon *m* médullaire
spinal cord (relating to); medullary médullaire *adj*
spinal cord inflammation; myelitis myélite *f*
spinal-cord nerve trapped by a slipped disc conflit *m* disco-radiculaire
spinal disc, of/concerning discal(e) *adj*
spinal meningitis méningite *f* cérébro-spinale

spinal nerve nerf *m* rachidien
spinal nerves nerfs *mpl* spinaux
spindly grêle *adj*
spine colonne *f* vertébrale
spit sputum *m*
splayed feet pieds *mpl* tournés en dehors
spleen rate *f*
spleen, oversized splénomégalie *f*
splenectomy (spleen removal) splénectomie *f*
splint appareil *m* pour fracture; attelle *f*; éclisse *f*
splints, to put in éclisser *v*
splinter écharde *f*
split nail ongle *m* dédoublé
spluttering (sound from lungs) sous-crépitant *adj*
spondylitis (inflammation of a vertebra) spondylite *f*
spondylopathy (spinal disease) spondylopathie *f*
sponge éponge *f*
spore (reproductive cell) spore *f*
spot (place) point *m*
spot bouton *m*
spot, beauty (mole) grain *m* de beauté *f*
spot, abnormally dark (on X-ray image) infiltrat *m*
spot, beauty; birthmark (harmless) naevus *m* simple
spot, beauty; birthmark (potentially cancerous) naevus naevocellulaire *m*
spot, multi-coloured (may be beginning of a cancer) tache *f* polychrome
spot (formed on healing cut/ wound) bourgeon *m*
spotty boutonneux -euse *adj*
sprain entorse *f*
sprain, serious (causing torn ligaments) entorse *f* grave
sprain, to fouler *v*
sprain one's ankle/wrist, to se fouler *v* la cheville / le poignet
sprained ankle entorse *f* à la chéville
sprained/strained back tour *m* de reins
sprained wrist entorse *f* au poignet
spray (aerosol) bombe *f* aerosol
spray (aerosol/vaporiser) pulvérisateur *m*
spraying pulvérisation *f*

spread, to (of illness) se généraliser *v*
spread an illness, to communiquer *v* une maladie
spreading invasif -ive *adj*; rayonnant(e) *adj*
sprue (tropical disease) sprue *f*
squama (scale) squame *f*
squamous squameux -euse *adj*
squint, to loucher *v*
stage phase *f*
stage (particularly of illness) période *f*; stade *m*
stairlift monte-escaliers *m*
stammering bégaiement *m*
standard-sized de dimension normale *f*
staphylococcia staphylococcie *f*
staphyloccus (bacterium, sometimes causing pus formation) staphylocoque *m*
staphyloccus aureus (grape-like formation) staphylocque *m* doré
starter culture ferment *m* lactique
stapes (small stirrup-shaped earbone) étrier *m*
start, to (treatment) instaurer *v*
stasis (stoppage/slowing down of circulation of any of the body fluids) stase *f*
state of shock, in a commotionné(e) *adj*
stay, to rester *v*
steam bath bain *m* de vapeur *f*; hammam *m*
steam inhalations, to use faire *v* des inhalations
steatopygy (fattiness in female buttocks) stéatopygie *f*
stenosis (abnormal narrowing of passage in body) sténose *f*
stent (metal tube used to widen arteries) stent *m*
stepping exercise machine stepper *m*
sterile stérile *adj*
sterile compress tricostéril *m*
sterility stérilité *f*
sterilise, to stériliser *v*
sterilise, to (with a flame) flamber *v*
sterilisation stérilisation *f*
sterilising solution solution de stérilisation *f*
sternum sternum *m*
steroid stéroïde *m*; lipide *m*

steroid hormone hydrocortisone *f*
steroidal hormone stéroïde *m* hormonal
stethoscope stéthoscope *m*
stethoscope examination auscultation *f* médiate
stick (cosmetics, cream, etc) stick *m*
stick in the throat, to rester *v* dans la gorge
stiffening or blockage (of muscle) enraidissement *m*
stiffness courbatures *f*; raideur *f*
stigma stigmate *m*
still-born baby enfant *m* mort-né(e) *m/f*
stimulate, to exciter *v*
sting piqûre *f*
sting, to piquer *v*
stinging nettle ortie *f* piquante
stirrup (mid-ear bone) étrier *m*
stitch point *m* de suture
stitch (ache) point *m* de côté
stitch back up, to (after operation) recoudre *v*
stitch up, to suturer *v*
St. John's wort (for infusions) millepertuis *m*
stock, to tenir *v*
stomach; abdomen abdomen *m*; estomac *m*; ventre *m*
stomach, excessive air in; aerogastria aérogastrie *f*
stomach, excess air in (temporary condition); aerophagy aérophagie *f*
stomach area, middle of épigastre *m*
stomach, of/concerning stomacal(e) *adj*; ventral(e) (*pl* -aux) *adj*
stomach ache douleur *f* abdominale; mal *m* à l'estomac
stomach bag operation stomie *m*
stomach cancer cancer *m* de l'estomac
stomach cramp crampe *f* d'estomac
stomach and digestive system disorders, study/treatment of: gastro-enterology gastro-entérologie *f* et appareil *m* digestif
stomach distension gonflement *m*
stomach investigation (opening) operation thoractomie *f*

stomach and lower stomach area étage *m* abdomino-pelvien
stomach area, lower (relating to) antral(e) *adj*
stomach muscles abdominaux *m*
stomach pump pompe *f* stomacale
stomach tube sonde *f* gastrique
stomach ulcer ulcère *f* à l'estomac
stomach ulcer medicine inhibiteur *m* de la pompe à protons
stomach upset embarras *m* gastrique; estomac *m* fatigué
stomach wash lavage *m* gastrique
stomach X-ray without prior treatment abdomen *m* sans préparation
stomatitis (mouth inflammation) stomatite *f*
stomatologist stomatologue *m/f*
stomatology (study of mouth and teeth or their diseases) stomatologie *f*
stone pierre *f*
stony pierreux -euse *adj*
stools selles *fpl*
stools sample prélèvement *m* de selles
stout build, of de forte corpulence *f*
stoutness corpulence *f*
strabismus (one or both eyes out of normal position) strabisme *m*
strain froissement *m*
strain, to (muscle) froisser *v*
strained fatigué(e) *adj*
strained/pulled (muscle) élongation *f*
strangulated hernia (blocking circulation) hernie *f* étranglée
strawberry mark fraise *f*; tache de naissance *f*; tache *f* de son de rousseur
streptococcus (bacterium) streptocoque *m*
streptococcus (causing scarlet fever, acute articular rheumatism) streptocoque *m* bêta-hémolytique
streptomycin (antibiotic) streptomycine *f*
stress stress *m*
stress, to put under stresser *v*
stressful stressant(e) *adj*
stretch mark vergeture *f*

stretcher brancard *m*; civière *f*
stretcher-bearer brancardier *m*
stretching (of muscle) extension *f*
stretching (of stomach) ballonnement *m*
stretching exercises stretching *m*
stricture (of canal/duct) rétrécissement *m*
strip off completely, to déshabiller *v* complètement
strip off to the waist, to déshabiller *v* jusqu'à la ceinture
stroke accident *m* vasculaire cérébral; congestion *f* cérébrale; ramollissement *m* cérébral
stroke lasting less than 24 hours accident *m* ischémique (cérébral)
stump (of limb) moignon *m*
stupefy, to stupéfier *v*
stupefying stupéfiant(e) *adj*
stupor stupeur *f*
sty(e) orgelet *m*
stylet (small probe) stylet *m*
sub-cutaneous injection injection sous-cutanée *f*
subsidence (fever) rémission *f*
sucking succion *f*
sucrose saccharose *m*
suction succion *f*
sudamina (heat spots) sudamina *m* (boutons *m* de chaleur *f*)
suffer, to souffrir *v*
suffering from atteint(e) *adj*
suffocation suffocation *f*; étouffement *m*
sugars, complex (slow) sucres *m* lents
sugar-coated pill dragée *f*
sugar-count equivalence between different quantities of different foods équivalence *f* glucidique
sugar-in-the-blood scale related to foods index *m* glucidique
suicide mort *f* volontaire; suicide *m*
sulphonamide (sulphonic acid derivative) sulfamide *m*
sun, of/concerning solaire *adj*
sun protection factor (on bottles, tubes etc.) indice *m* de protection *f* solaire
sun screen (cream) écran *m* solaire
sunbathing bains *mpl* de soleil

sunbathing, body's capacity to resist long-term harmful effects of capital soleil *m*
sunbed sessions, to have faire *v* des séances *fpl* d'ultraviolets
sunblock, total (cream/lotion) écran *m* total
sunburn coup *m* de soleil
sunglasses lunettes *fpl* de soleil
sunstroke insolation *f*
suntan cream crème *f* solaire
suntan emulsion émulsion *f* solaire
suntan lotion crème *f* solaire; lotion *f* solaire
suntan oil huile *f* solaire
suntan spray spray *m* solaire
suntanning bronzage *m*
suppleness compliance *f*
support/appliance enabling limb to function orthèse *f*
support bandage strapping *m*
support, strong (includes plasters, support stockings and splints) contention *f*
suppository suppositoire *m*
suppurate, to suppurer *v*
suppuration (formation of pus) suppuration *f*
surgeon chirurgien(ne) *m/f*
surgery (incl. manual and laser) chirurgie *f*
surgery (premises) cabinet *m* médical
surgery, computer-aided (surgetics) surgetique *f*
surgery to the hand chirurgie *f* de la main
surgery to the urinary system chirurgie urologique *f*
surgery treating but conserving breast affected by breast cancer chirurgie *f* conservatrice du cancer *m* du sein
surgetics (computer-aided surgery) surgetique *f*
surgical appliance bandage *m* herniaire
surgical clip agrafe *f*
surgical collar minerve *f*
surgical corset ceinture *f* orthopédique
surgical cotton wool/cotton ouate *f* chirurgicale
surgical cotton for wound drainage séton *m* à mèche
surgical incision (into skin or organ) solution de continuité *f*

surgical introduction of a cannula tubage *m*
surgical mask masque *m* chirurgical
surgical metal plate plaque *f*
surgical operation intervention *f* chirurgicale
surgical knife lancette *f*
surgical scalpel bistouri *m*
surgical smoothening of the skin abrasion *f*
surgical spirits alcool à 90 *m*
surrogate mother (illegal in France) mère *f* porteuse
susceptibility réceptivité *f*
sustain, to (with food) sustenter *v*
suture point *m* de suture
suture (thread) suture *f*
suture, to suturer *v*
swab tampon *m*
swallow, to avaler *v*; déglutir *v*
swallowing déglutition *f*
swallowing, difficulty in dysphagie *f*
sweat, to come out in a/to break into a piquer *v* une suée *f*
sweat sueur *f*; sudation *f*; perspiration *f*
sweat gland glande *f* sudoripaire
sweat glands, inflammation of hydrosadénite *f*
sweating, excessive; hyperhidrosis hyperhidrose *f*
sweet clover mélilot *m*
sweet diabetes diabète *m* sucré
sweetener édulcorant *m*
sweetener, artificial édulcorant *m* de synthèse
swell, to enfler *v*
swell up, to enfler *v*; gonfler *v*
swell up again, to regonfler *v*
swelling bombement *f* (esp. forehead); enflure *f*; fluxion *f*; gonflement *m*
swelling, small; nodule nodule *m*
swimming natation *f*
swimming goggles lunettes *fpl* de natation
swollen bladder, shape of globe *m* vésical
swollen glands, to have avoir *v* des ganglions *mpl*
swollen visible blood vessels; acne rosacea acné *f* rosacée
St Vitus's dance danse *f* de St Guy

sycosis (facial disease in bearded area) sycosis *m*
Sydenham's chorea chorée *f*
symptom (change felt by patient) symptôme *m*
symptoms and consequences of infection processus *m* infectieux
synapse (neurotransmission gap between two nerve cells) synapse *f*
syndrome syndrome *m*
synergy synergie *f*
synergist (medicine or organ working with another) synergiste *m*
synergistic synergiste *adj*
synovial fluid/liquid (lubricates joints and tendon sheathes) liquide *m* synovial
synovial membrane (around joints) synoviale *f*
synovitis (inflammation of the synovial membrane) synovite *f*
syphilis syphilis *f*
syringe seringue *f*
syringe tips, single-use embouts *mpl* jetables de seringues
system système *m*
systemic systémique *adj*
systemic illness (term for a number of illnesses which spread throughout the body, but with little known origin) maladie *f* systémique
systemic infection (throughout the whole body) infection *f* généralisée
systole (intervals between heart contractions when blood is pumped into arteries) systole *f*
systolic blood pressure tension *f* artérielle systolique

t'ai chi Tai-chi-chuan *m*; Tai-ji-quan *m*
tablespoonful cuillérée *f* à soupe
tablet (aspirin, vitamin, etc.) comprimé *m*
tablet, chewable cachet *m* à croquer
tablet, coated comprimé *m* pelliculé

tablet form sous forme *f* de comprimés

tablet taken under the tongue comprimé *m* sublingual; linguette *f*

tachyarrythmia (irregular heartbeat with fast bursts) tachyarythmie *f*

tachycardia (abnormally fast heart rate) tachycardie *f*

taenia (tapeworm) ténia *m*; taenia *m*

take, to (medicine etc.) prendre *v*

take a sample, to prélever *v* un échantillon *m*

talcum powder talc *m*

talus (ankle bone supporting tibia) astragale *m*

tampon tampon hygiènique *m*

tamponade; tamponage (compression of the heart disorder) tamponnement *m*

tap, to tapoter *v*

tapeworm ténia *m*; taenia *m*; ver solitaire *m*

tapotement (percussion massage) tapotement *m*

tarsal bone os *m* du tarse

tarsus (the group of ankle and upper foot bones) tarse *m*

tartar tartre *m*

taste goût *m*

taste bud papille de la langue *f*; papille linguale *f*; papille gustative *f*

tattoo tatouage *m*

tattooing tatouage *m*

TB microbe bacille *f* de Koch

TB vaccine vaccin *m* contre la tuberculose

tear (eye) larme *f*

tear (laceration) déchirure *f*

tear, to déchirer *v*

tear a muscle, to se déchirer *v* un muscle

tear duct voie lacrymale *f*; canal lacrymal *m*

tears (eye) liquide lacrymal *m*; larmes *fpl*

tears (eye), of/concerning lachrymal(e) (*pl* -aux) *adj*

teaspoonful cuillérée *f* à café

teat (baby's bottle) tétine *f*

teeth dents *fpl*

teeth, back dents *fpl* du fond; dents *fpl* de derrière

teeth, false fausses dents *m*

teeth, front dents *f* de devant

teeth, lower dents *f* du bas
teeth, set of denture *f*
teeth, upper dents *f* du haut
teeth, clenching/grinding of; bruxism mâchonnement *m*
teeth, X-ray of all panoramique dentaire *m*
teeth brace appareil *m* orthodontique; appareil *m* de contention dentaire
teeth straightening orthodontie *f*
teething poussées dentaires *fpl*; poussée de dents *f*
teething ring anneau *m* de dentition
tegument (skin, body hair) tegument *m*
telecobalt machine bombe *f* au cobalt *m*
teleradiography (X-rays from a certain distance for increased precision) téléradiographie *f*
teleradiotherapy téléradiothérapie *f*
temporal (temple) bone temporal *m*
temperature température *f*
temperature, high fièvre *f*
temperature, slight fébricule *f*
temperature, to have a avoir/faire *v* de la température
temperature, to take (someone's) prendre *v* la température
temperature chart feuille de température *f*
temple tempe *f*
tendinitis (inflammation of the tendon) enthésiopathie *f*; tendinite *f*
tendon tendon *m*
tennis elbow épicondylite *f*
tent (lint/linen inserted into a wound) mèche *f*
teratogenic (of illnesses/medicines suffered/taken in early pregnancy which can produce malformation in babies) tératogène *adj*
term terme *m*
terminally-ill patient malade *m/f* condamné(e)
terminate, to interrompre *v*
termination of pregnancy (voluntary) interruption *f* voluntaire de grossesse (IVG)

termination of pregnancy (for medical reasons) avortement *m* thérapeutique
tertiary tertiaire *adj*
test épreuve *f*
testicle testicule *m*
testicle or ovary; gonad gonade *f*
testicle inflammation; orchitis orchite *f*
testosterone (male hormone) testostérone *f*
tetanus tétanos *m*
(anti-)tetanus vaccine vaccin *m* contre le tétanos
tetany (muscle spasm) tétanie *f*
tetracycline (type of antibiotic) tétracycline *f*
tetraplegic (person with total limb paralysis); quadraplegic tétraplégique *m/f*
thalamus (darker tissues of forebrain) thalamus *m*
thalassemia (illness at birth due to lack of red corpuscles) thalassémie *f*
thalassotherapy (sea-water therapy) thalassothérapie *f*
therapeutic therapeutique *adj*
therapeutic effectiveness efficacité *f* thérapeutique
therapeutic medicine agent *m* thérapeutique
therapeutic properties propriétés *m* thérapeutiques
therapeutics thérapeutique *f*
therapeutics/treatments (classed as alternative/non-conventional medicine) thérapeutiques *fpl* diverses
thermal compression moulding (chiropodist's false soles, etc.) thermoformage *f*
thermal water eau *f* thermale
thermometer thermomètre *m*
thermometer, alcohol thermomètre *m* à alcool
thermometer, clinical thermomètre *m* clinique
thermometer, electronic thermomètre *m* électronique
thermometer, infrared thermomètre *m* à infrarouges
thermometer, maximum and minimum thermomètre *m* à maxima et minima
thermometer, mercury thermomètre *m* à mercure

thermotherapy (heat treatment) thermotherapie *f*
thickener, instant (for thickening food) poudre *f* épaississante
thigh cuisse *f*
thigh, of/concerning crural(e) *adj*
thigh nerve nerf *m* crural
thigh pain cruralgie *f*
thin maigre *adj*
thinness maigreur *m* (see also indice de masse corporelle in French-English section)
third degree burn brûlure *f* du troisième degré
thirst soif *f*
thoracic/rib cage cage *f* thoracique
thoracic duct canal *m* thoracique
thorax thorax *m*
thorax and lung membranes, of/concerning; pleura pleural(e) (*pl* -aux) *adj*
threadworm oxyure *m*
three complementary medicines as treatment trithérapie *f*
throat gorge *f*
throat, hoarse gorge *f* prise
throat, sore mal *m* à la gorge
throat cancer cancer *m* de l'oesphage
throat infection angine *f*
throat infection, back and bottom of the angine *f* pharyngienne
throat pastilles pastilles *fpl* pour la gorge
throbbing palpitant(e) *adj*
throbbing pain douleur *f* lancinante
thrombin (causes blood clotting) thrombine *f*
thrombosis thrombose *f*
throwaway razor rasoir *m* jetable
thrush (white patchy infection of the mouth and throat and/or the vagina) candidose *f*; moniliase *f*
thumb pouce *f*
thymic (of/concerning the thymus) thymique *adj*
thymus (neck gland) thymus *m*
thyroid thyroïde *adj*
thyroid gland glande *f* thyroïde

thyroid gland, subnormal activity of; hypothyroidism hypothyroïdie *f*

tibia (shin bone) tibia *m*

tic tic *m*

ticker (heart) palpitant *m* (informal)

tie up, to ligaturer *v*

tincture of arnica teinture *f* d'arnica; teinture *f* d'iodine

tinea (ringworm) teigne *f*

tinnitus (ringing in ears) acouphène *m*

tip (finger, nose etc.) bout *m*

tip (point) pointe *f*

tire, to fatiguer *v*

tired fatigué(e) *adj*

tired, to get fatiguer *v*

tissue (paper) mouchoir en papier *m*

tissue (body) tissu *m*

tissue, connective tissu *m* conjonctif

tissue formation, new néoformation *f*

tissue growth, new abnormal (or tumour) néoplasme *m*

tissue group (type) groupe *m* tissulaire

titanium (used in prostheses) titane *m*

toadstool champignon *m* vénéneux

tobacco poisoning intoxication *f* tabagique

tobacco use, of/concerning tabagique *adj*

toe orteil *m*; doigt de pied *m*

toe, big gros orteil *m*

toe, little petit orteil *m*

toenail ongle de l'orteil *m*; ongle du pied *m*

toilets toilettes *fpl*; cabinets *mpl*

toilet paper papier *m* hygiènique; papier *m* toilette

toilet soap savon *m* de toilette

tolerance (to treatment or to receptivity of graft) tolérance *f*

tolerate, to tolérer *v*

tomography (3D medical imagery/scanning) tomographie *f*

tongue langue *f*

tongue, coated/furred langue *f* blanche/chargée/pâteuse

tongue, of/concerning lingual(e) (*pl* -aux) *adj*

tongue out, to put the tirer *v* la langue
tongue, putting out the protraction *f* linguale
tonic remontant *m*; tonique *m*
tonicity tonicité *f*
tonsil tonsille *f*
tonsillectomy (surgical removal of tonsils) amygdalectomie *f*
tonsillitis amygdalite *f*; angine rouge *f*; tonsillite *f*
tonsils amygdales *fpl*
tooth dent *f*
tooth, artificial dent *f* artificielle
tooth, bad dent *f* gâtée
tooth, canine canine *f*
tooth, capping of; crown couronne *f* dentaire
tooth, decayed dent *f* cariée
tooth, filled dent *f* obturée
tooth, hollow dent *f* creuse
tooth, milk (baby) dent *f* de lait
tooth, wisdom dent *f* de sagesse
tooth, second (permanent) dent *f* définitive; dent *f* de remplacement
tooth decay carie *f*
tooth extraction avulsion *f* dentaire
tooth powder poudre *f* dentifrice
tooth root racine *f* nerveuse
toothache mal *m* aux dents
toothache, to have avoir *v* mal aux dents
toothbrush brosse *f* à dents
toothpaste dentifrice *m*
toothpaste, fluoride dentifrice *m* fluoré
toothpick cure-dents *m*
topical/local (medicine/pain/ anaesthetic) topique *m* and *adj*
torsion torsion *f*
torticollis (**wry/stiff neck**) torticolis *m*
touch (massage) lightly, to effleurer *v*
touch, sense of toucher *m*
tourist's diarrhoea tourista *f*
tourniquet garrot *m*; tourniquet *m*
toxaemia toxémie *f*
toxic toxique *adj*
toxic shock choc *m* septique
Toxic Shock Syndrome (TSS) syndrome du choc toxique *m*; SCT

toxicologist (poison specialist) toxicologue *m/f*
toxicology toxicologie *f*
toxin toxine *f*
toxiplasmosis (parasitical infection) toxoplasmose f
tracaganth (white/reddish pharmaceutical gum dye) gomme *f* adragante
trace element (for normal growth) oligoélément *m*
tracer (radioactive isotope trace in medical imagery) marqueur *m*
tracheal (**of/concerning windpipe)** tracheal(e) (*pl* -aux) *adj*
tracheotomy trachéotomie *f*; intubation trachéale *f*
trachoma (eye infection) trachome *m*
tract (area of an organ or body system) tractus *m*
tract (duct) voie *f*
traction (limb) traction *f*; extension *f*
trance catalepsie *f*
tranquilliser anxiolytique *m*; tranquillisant *m*
tranquillising anxiolytique *adj*; tranquillisant(e) *adj*
transfuse, to transfuser
transfusion transfusion *f*
transgenic (such as foodstuff with genetically modified animal or vegetable content) transgénique *adj*
transmit (illness), to transmettre *v*
transplant greffe *f*
transplant, to greffer *v*; transplanter *v*
transplantation transplantation *f*
transport transplantation *f*
transport of person in accident to hospital évacuation *f*
trauma trauma *m*
trauma, cranial traumatisme *m* crânien
traumatic traumatique *adj*
traumatism traumatisme *m*
travel sickness mal *m* des transports
treadmill exerciser tapis *m* roulant
treat, to traiter *v*
treat illness/patient, to soigner *v*

treatment soins *mpl*; thérapeutique *f*; traitement *m*
treatment, current methods of moyens *m* thérapeutiques actuels
treatment, secondary (additional to the essential treatment) traitement *m* adjuvant
treatment, sustaining traitement d'entretien *m*
treatment for alcoholism cure *f* de désintoxication *f*
treatment (preparation) prior to investigation or surgery préparation *f*
treatment before check-up to give real state of health, to stop démaquiller *v*
treatment not stopped sufficienftly in advance of examination for a true result traitement *m* maquillé
treatment through antibiotics antibiothérapie *f*
treatment using two medicines bithérapie *f*
tremble, to trembler *v*
trembling tremblement *m*
tremor trémulation *f*
trepanation (surgical opening of bone, esp. skull) trépanation *f*
trepanation, surgical bore for trépan *m*
trial épreuve *f*
triceps triceps *m*
triceps saural (the two calf muscles) jumeaux *mpl*
triglyceride (fat compounds in the blood) triglycéride *m*
trisomy 21 (Down's syndrome) trisomie *f* 21
tropical disease maladie *f* tropicale
trunk tronc *m*
truss bandage *m* herniaire
tube, short pharmaceutical packaging bâtonnet *m*
tubal (relating to Fallopian tube) tubaire *adj*
tubercle (small rounded protuberance or swelling) tubercule *m*
tubercular; tuberculous tuberculeux -euse *adj*
tuberculosis tuberculose *f*
tumefaction tuméfaction *f*

tummy, to have a/to be getting a avoir/prendre *v* du ventre *m*
tumour tumeur *f*; néoformation *f*
tumour/growth (benign) adénome *m*
tumour (benign) near genitals condylome *m*
tumour, brain astrocytome *f*
tumour, brain or nerve gliome *m*
tumour, surgical operation to remove ablation *f*; exérèse *f*
tumour (benign) near genitals, sexually transmitted condylome *m* acuminé
tweezers (for removing splinters) pince *f* à échardes
twin jumeau *m* -elle *f*
twins jumeaux *m* -elles *f*
twist/sprain one's ankle/wrist, to se fouler *v* la cheville *f*/le poignet *m*
twisted (blocked) intestine; volvulus volvulus *m*
typhoid typhoïde *f*
typhoid fever fièvre *f* typhoïde
typhus typhus *m*
ulcer ulcère *m*
ulcerate, to ulcérer *v*
ulcerated ulcéreux -euse *adj*
ulceration ulcération *f*
ulna (forearm bone) cubitus *m*
ultrasonic ultrasonique *adj*
ultrasound heart scan échocardiographie *f*
ultrasound scan échographie *f* (abbrev. écho *f*)
ultrasound (scans) ultrason *m*
ultrasound scan image échographie *f*
ultrasound scanner échographe *m*
ultraviolet ultraviolet -ette *adj*
ultraviolet radiation rayonnement *m* ultraviolet
umbilical cord cordon *m* ombilical
umbilicus nombril *m*; ombilic *m*
unbandage, to débander *v*
unblock, to libérer *v*
unconscious évanoui(e) *adj*
unconsciousness, loss of perte de connaissance *f*
uncovered body area, ready for surgery champ *m* opératoire
undulant fever brucellose *f*

underarm crutch béquille *f* commune
undergo therapy, to faire *v* de la rééducation *f*
undernourishment, moderate (10–15 per cent weight loss) dénutrition *f* modérée
undernourishment, severe (over 15 per cent weight loss) dénutrition *f* sévère
undernourishment, slight (5–10 per cent weight loss) dénutrition *f* légère
underweight maigre *adj* (see also indice de masse corporelle in French-English section)
unharmed indemne *adj*
unit unité f
universal recipient receveur -euse *m/f* universel(lle) *m/f*
unpasteurised milk lait *m* cru
unstable (condition) instable *adj*
unstable (products, mood, condition) labile *adj*
unweaned baby nourrisson *m*
unwell souffrant(e) *adj*
'up'side (of artery: to stem bleeding) en amont
upset embarras *m*
upset stomach embarras *m* gastrique
uraemia (raised blood level in nitrogeneous waste compounds) urémie *f*
urea (nitrogenous compound in urine) urée *f*
ureter (urine canal from kidney to bladder) uretère *m*
ureteral (of/concerning the ureter) urétéral(e) (*pl* -aux) *adj*
urethra (urine discharge duct from the bladder) urètre *m*
urethral (of/concerning the uretha) urétral(e) (*pl* -aux) *adj*
urethral tube sonde *f* urétrale
uric acid acide *m* urique
uric acid level in blood uricémie *f*
urinary bladder vessie *f*
urinary tract voies *f* urinaire
urinary tract stones; gravel gravelle *f*
urination miction *f*
urination, abnormal increase in amounts of polyurie *f*
urination, frequent (in small amounts); pollakurie pollakiurie *f*

urination, painful/difficult; dysuria dysurie *f*
urination capacity reduction; oliguria oligurie *f*
urine urine *f*
urine, abnormal protein count in; albuminuria albuminurie *f*
urine in full bladder, measured amount of volumétrie *f* vésicale prémictionnelle
urine outlet in male and female genitals méat *m* urinaire
urine reflux from bladder to kidneys reflux *m* vésico-urétéral
urine sample prélèvement *m* d'urine
urine test analyse *f* d'urine
urogenital urogénital(e) (*pl* -aux) *adj*
urogenital system appareil *m* urogénital
urology (study of the urinary system) urologie *f*
urticaria (nettle rash or hives) urticaire *f*
use before (e.g. on medicines) à utiliser avant (abbrev. à ut. av.)
use, for external/internal à usage *m* externe/interne
uterus matrice *f*; utérus *m*
uterus displacement déviation *f* de l'utérus
uveal tract (pigmented layer of the eye) uvée *f*
uvula (fleshy extension of soft palate hanging above throat) luette *f*

vaccinate, to vacciner *v*
vaccination vaccination *f*
vaccination, to have a se faire *v* vacciner *v*
vaccine vaccin *m*
vaccine, diphtheria/tetanus/poliomyelitis vaccin *m* contre la diphtérie/le tétanos/poliomyélite
vaccine with several different functions vaccine *m* polyvalent
vagal (relating to vagus: a cranial nerve) vagal(e) *adj*
vagal nerve surgery vagotomie *f*
vagina vagin *m*

vagina, inflammation of vaginité *f*
vagina, through the (for administration of medicine)par voie *f* transvaginale
vaginal vaginal(e) (*pl* -aux) *adj*
vaginal contraceptive device préservatif *m* (féminin)
vaginal douche douche *f* vaginale; lavage *m* interne
vaginal discharge; leucorrhea pertes *fpl* blanches
vaginal finger probe toucher *m* vaginal
vaginal flora (not abnormal) flore *f* vaginale
vaginal suppository ovule *m* (pharmacie); pessaire *m*
vaginal thrush (infection) mycose *f* vaginale
vagus nerve (cranial nerve) nerf *f* vague
valerian (sedative) valériane *f*
valve valve *f*
valve, heart valve *f* cardiaque
valve allowing blood flow in one direction valvule *f*
vaporiser pulvérisateur *m*
varicose ulcer ulcère *m* variqueux
varicose vein; varix varice *f*
varicose-vein operation as outpatient cure *f* conservatrice et hyémodynamique de l'insuffisance veineuse en ambulatoire (CHIVA)
varicose vein removal stripping *m*; éveinage *m*
vas deferens (spermatic duct from testicle to uretha) canal *m* déférent
vascular (blood vessel) surgery chirurgie *f* vasculaire
vasectomy vasectomie *f*
vaseline ® vaseline ® *f*
vasoconstriction vasoconstriction *f*
vasoconstrictor (agent causing constriction of blood vessels) vasoconstricteur *m*
vasoconstrictive (causing constriction of blood vessels) vasoconstricteur -trice *adj*
vasodilation vasodilatation *f*

vasodilating (causing dilatation of blood vessels) vasodilateur -trice *adj*

vault of the cranium voûte *f* crânienne

VD groin ulcer chancre *m* mou; chancrelle *f*

vegan végétalien(ne) *adj*

veganism végétalisme *m*

vegetarian végétarien(ne) *adj*

vegetarianism végétarisme *m*

vein veine *f*

vein, surgical repair of impaired angioplastie *f*

vein inflammation; phlebitis phlébite *f*

vein removal éveinage *m*; stripping *m*

vein specialist phlébologue *f*

veins and arteries, X-rays of; angiography angiographie *f*

vena cava (into the heart) veine cave *f*

venereal vénérien(ne) *adj*

venereal disease (VD) maladie honteuse/vénérienne *f*

venereology vénéréologie *f*

venom venin *m*

venomous venimeux -euse *adj*

venomous bite morsure *f* venimeuse

venous veineux -euse *adj*

ventilate, to (oxygenate the blood or admit/propel air into the lungs) ventiler *v*

ventilation ventilation *f*

ventilation, artificial ventilation *f* artificielle

ventilation, assisted respiration *f* assistée

Ventoline ® (spray, syrup, or ampoule injection to counter asthma) Ventoline ® *f*

ventricle (body cavity or organ hollow) ventricule *m*

ventricular fibrillation fibrillation *f* ventriculaire *f* (FV)

verbal fluency fluence *f* verbale

verbal prescription prescription *f*

vermifuge (expels intestinal worms) vermifuge *m*

verruca verrue *f* plantaire

vertebra (*pl* -ae) vertèbre *f*

vertebral vertébral(e) (*pl* -aux) *adj*

vertebral column; spine colonne *f* vertébrale; colonne *f* rachidienne; rachis *m*
vertebrate vertébré *m*
vertex (crown of the head) vertex *m*
vertiginous vertigineux -euse *adj*
vertigo vertige *m*
vertigo, to suffer from avoir *v* des vertiges
very small amount (biology) trace *f*
vesicatory (eruption of blisters) vésicatoire *m*
vesicatory (eruption of blisters) vésicatoire *adj*
vesicle (fluid filled sac/cyst/ blister) vésicule *f*
vesicles, seminal vésicules *fpl* séminales
vestibule (channel/chamber leading to another) vestibule *m*
vibrations vibrations *fpl*
vibrator vibromasseur *m*
Vincent's angina (pectoris) angine *f* de Vincent
viral hepatitis hépatite *f* virale
viral pneumonia pneumonie *f* virale
viral throat infection angine *f* virale
virilism (abnormal development of secondary male characteristics) virilisation *f*
virology (study of viruses) virologie *f*
virology laboratory laboratoire de viriologie *f*
virus virus *m*
virus in the blood virémie *f*
virus count in blood charge *f* virale
viscera (organs) viscères *mpl*
visceral viscéral(e) (*pl* -aux) *adj*
visceral surgery (to principal body organs) chirurgie *f* viscérale
visible, to make (using med. equipment) visualiser *v*
vision vision *f*
vision, double vision *f* double
vision, field of champ *m* visual
vision/sight, line of rayon *m* de vision
vision (view) vue *f*

visual hallucination hallucination *f* visuelle
visually handicapped person déficient(e) *m/f* visuel(le) *f*
vitaliser vitaliseur *m*
vitality vitalité *f*
vitality rating (of newborn baby); Apgar index indice *m* d'Apgar
vitamin vitamine *f*
vitamin B; riboflavin riboflavine *f*
vitamin deficiency carence *f* en vitamines
vitamin-deficiency illness avitaminose *f*
vitamin-enriched milk lait *m* de croissance
vitamin tablet/pill comprimé *m* de vitamines
vitamins, with added vitaminé(e) *adj*
vitiligo (skin de-pigmentation) vitiligo *m*
vitreous body (eye) corps *m* vitré
vitreous humour/body (clear tissue behind eyeball lens) humeur *f* vitreuse
vocal cord corde *f* vocale
vocal organs appareil *m* phonatoire
voice, temporary loss of aphonie *f*
volvulus (twisted/blocked intestine) volvulus *m*
vomit vomi *m*
vomiting vomissement *m*
vomit, to vomir *v*
vulva vulve *f*
vulva and vagina inflammation vilvo-vaginite *f*
vulvitis (vulva inflammation) vulvite *f*

waist taille *f*
walking frame déambulateur *m*
walking stick canne *f*
wall (anatomical) paroi *m*
wan, to look avoir *v* une petite mine *f*
wandering, aimlessly (of mentally ill) déambulation *f*
ward salle *f* d'hôpital *m*; service *m*; unité *f*
warming balm baume *m* chauffant
warning mise en garde *f*
wart papillome *m*; verrue *f*
wash out, to laver *v*

washing lavage *m*
washing out lavage *m*
washrooms sanitaires *mpl*
wasp sting piqûre de guêpe *f*
waste away, to se nécroser *v*
wasting disease maladie *f* de langeur
water eau *f*, eaux (*fpl*)
water, drinking (outside/ fountains etc.) eau *f* potable
water, mineral eau *f* minérale
water, non-drinking eau *f* non potable
water, spring eau *f* de source
water, tap eau *f* du robinet (eau municipale *f*)
waters have broken, her elle a perdu *v* les eaux
water bed lit *m* d'eau
water cures thermalisme *m*
water on the knee épanchement *m* de synovie
waterproof étanche *adj*
waterproof chair for the bath siège de bain *m*
water-swollen kidney; hydronephosis hydronéphrose *f*
wax cire *f*; lipide *m*
WC water-closet *m*; WC *m*
weak faible *adj*
weaning sevrage *m*
wearing away/erosion of the invertebrate disc discarthrose *f*
weary fatigué(e) *adj*
weighing scales pèse-bébé *m*
weighing scales, bathroom pèse-personne *m*
weighing scales with dial pèse-personne *m* à cadran aiguille
weighing scales with digital reading pèse-personne *m* digital
weight poids *m*
weight, excess (too much for good health) surcharge *f* pondérale
weight loss perte *f* de poids
wen (benign skin tumour) kyste sébacé *m*; loupe *f*
wet dreams (spontaneous ejaculation during sleep) pollutions *fpl* nocturnes
wheatgerm germes *mpl* de blé
wheelchair fauteuil *m* roulant
wheelchair with reclining back fauteuil *m* roulant à dossier inclinable

wheezing respiration *f* bruyante/sifflante

whistling sibilant(e) *adj*

whistling sound in ears sifflement *m*

white corpuscle; leucocyte globule *m* blanc; leucocyte *m*

white corpuscles, abnormal reduction in agranulocytose *f*

white of the eye; sclera sclérotique *f*

white stick canne *f* blanche

whitish-grey liquid patch forming on eye arc *m* lipoïdique

whitish throat infection angine *f* blanche

whitlow (inflammation next to nail) panaris *m*

whistling sounds in ear; tinnitus acouphène *m*

whooping cough coqueluche *f*

(anti-) whooping cough vaccine vaccin *m* contre la coqueluche

wick (gauze strip for wounds) mèche *f*

widening of bronchial tubes bronchectasie *f*

wig perruque *f*

willpower, loss of; aboulia aboulie *f*

wind flatuosité *f*

windpipe trachée-artère *f*; trachée *f*

windpipe, of/concerning; tracheal tracheal(e) (*pl* -aux) *adj*

windpipe and alimentary canal, cross-over junction between carrefour *m* laryngé

windpipe inflammation trachéite *f*

wipes, baby lingettes *fpl* de bébé

witch-hazel hamamélis *m*

withdrawal symptoms symptômes *mpl* de sevrage

Wolff-Parkinson-White syndrome (sudden bursts of rapid heartbeats) syndrome *m* de Wolff-Parkinson-White

woman who has never been pregnant; nulligest nulligeste *f*

womb matrice *f*; utérus *m*

womb, descent of prolapsus *m* utérin

womb cancer cancer *m* du col de l'utérus

womb-muscle tumour myome *m* utérin
womb X-ray; hysterography hystérographie *f*
wooden leg jambe *f* de bois
work hygiene hygiène *f* du travail
working fonctionnement *m*
'worms', bilharzia bilharziose *f*; schistosomiase *f*
worsening nature (of illness) évolutivité *f*
wound blessure *f*; plaie *f*
wound, gaping blessure *f* béante
wound, to blesser *v*
wound oneself, to se blesser
wrinkle ride *f*
wrist poignet *m*
wrist bone; carpus os *m* du carpe *m*
wrist bones, of/concerning intercarpien(ne) *adj*
wrist plaster (cast) manchette *f* plâtrée
writer's cramp crampe *f* de l'écrivain *m*
written prescription ordonnance *f*
wrong way (of food/drink going down the 'wrong way') fausse route *f*
wry/stiff neck; torticollis torticolis *m*

xanthoma (skin disease) xanthome *m*
xiphoid process (cartilage below the sternum) processus *m* xiphoïde
X-ray cliché *m*
X-ray department service *m* radiologique
X-ray, to radiographier *v*
X-ray image, abnormal dark spot on infiltrat *m*
X-ray of arteries artériographie *f*
X-ray of coronary arteries coronarographie *f*
X-ray or other radiation examination examen *m* radiographique
X-ray of all teeth panoramique *m* dentaire
X-ray result (picture, plate on film) radiographie *f*; radio (abbrev.) *f*
X-ray taken, to have an passer *v* une radiographie/radio *f*

X-rays radiographie *f*; radio (abbrev.) *f*

yaws (contagious tropical disease) pian *m*
yellow body (hormone-secreting structure developed in ovary) corps *m* jaune
yellow fever fièvre *f* jaune
yellow melilot mélilot *m*
yoga yoga *m*

zimmer frame déambulateur *m*
zygomatic zygomatique *adj*
zygomatic arch (prominent cheek bone) arcade *f* zygomatique
zygote (cell formed by union of two sexual reproduction cells) zygote *m*

DICTIONARY

FRENCH BUILDING TERMS

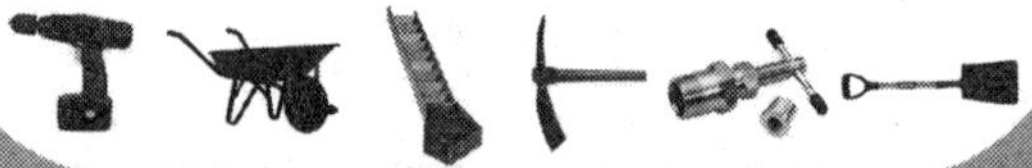

ESSENTIAL FOR RENOVATORS AND HOME-OWNERS

FRENCH – ENGLISH
ENGLISH – FRENCH

summersdale

Dictionary of French Building Terms
Essential for Renovators and Home-Owners

Richard Wiles

£12.99 Pb

ISBN: 1-84024-494-1

ISBN 13: 978-1-84024-494-6

Whether you own a home or work in France, this book will help you to communicate with French tradesmen.

- Accessible and comprehensive, the most up-to-date and easy-to-use dictionary of French building terms
- English–French and French–English
- Includes hundreds of technical words you won't find in an ordinary dictionary
- Will help you to avoid costly misunderstandings
- Covers tools and equipment for every aspect of carpentry, construction, decorating, ironmongery, metalwork, plumbing and heating
- Also includes terminology for financial and property matters, and an appendix of useful phrases

Editor Richard Wiles is an expert on home renovation, DIY and interior design. He is a translator and has written and edited over a dozen books on home improvement and France. He has contributed to *Living France* and *Everything France*, and produced *Successful DIY*, an English language version of the French *Guide Pratique du Bricolage*.

'If you've just returned from a fortnight in France with dreams of owning a property there, the Dictionary Of French Building Terms: Essential For Renovators And Homeowners, by Richard Wiles, could provide some of the practical know-how to turn your pie-in-the-sky scheme into reality.' The Mail on Sunday

'This is what we have been waiting for.' Living France magazine

'With hundreds of words you wouldn't find in a standard French dictionary, this guide will help you avoid potentially expensive misunderstandings...'
Destination France

www.summersdale.com